D0602476

GUT HEALTHY
COOKBOOK

Publications International, Ltd.

CONTENTS

INTRODUCTION

Eating and drinking are often taken for granted. Normally the human body's digestive system digests and metabolizes everything we eat and drink for energy or storage and the rest is eliminated. That is, unless there are snags along the pathway such as food allergies, intolerances or sensitivities, or a problematic gastrointestinal (GI) tract.

By understanding what happens to every mouthful, you may be able to appreciate your next bite or swallow and think about how to treat your GI tract (aka "gut") for maximal performance and health.

Good nutrition begins and depends upon effective digestion, absorption, and metabolism of nutrients. For people with gut problems, you'll find clarity in how to manage GI disorders for better nutrition and health.

Digestion and Gut Health

Digestion is the process by which foods and beverages are physically and chemically altered into smaller components by the human body that are then absorbed, metabolized for energy, or stored for future use.

During each stage of the digestive process (oral cavity, stomach, small, and large intestines), the macronutrients carbohydrates, fats, and proteins are broken down into their building blocks.

Along with vitamins, minerals, and water these building blocks are then used to fuel the body, build or rebuild it, protect the body from disease, rebound from illnesses, and a host of other functions.

What is not utilized is stored in forms that the body may be able to tap if and when necessary. All of these functions depend upon healthy digestion.

Sensory Stimuli

Digestion is activated by reactions to sensory stimuli. *Sensory stimuli* (how foods and beverages look, smell, and even sound) inform and protect the human body and trigger digestive juices "to flow".

Foods or beverages that are perceived as tasty may pleasantly stimulate the central nervous system, while foods or beverages that are perceived as offensive may have adverse effects.

Then chemical messengers in the oral cavity and GI tract transmit this information to the brain that triggers salivation and readies the body for digestion.

Normal digestion

Normal digestion may take from 24 to 48, even up to 72 hours depending upon the composition of foods and beverages.

By and large, the more components of a food or beverage, the more challenging it is for the body to handle. Carbohydrates tend to take the shortest amount of time for digestion (sugars in soft drinks may take as little as 15 minutes, and starches in pasta may take upwards of 2 to 3 hours).

A skinless chicken breast may take 5 to 6 hours to fully digest its protein, a cup of fruit juice may digest faster than a piece of fruit because of its higher fiber composition, and butter with its saturated fat content may need about 9 to 12 hours to complete digestion.

Oral Cavity

Chemical and physical digestion starts in the *oral cavity.* The oral cavity includes the lips, inside lining of the lips and cheeks, teeth, gums, front two-thirds of the tongue, floor of the mouth below the tongue, and the bony roof of the mouth.

In *chemical digestion,* digestive enzymes such as *salivary amylase* are released by the salivary glands to begin the chemical digestive process. In *physical digestion* the teeth and tongue help to break down, moisten, and move foods to the back of the oral cavity for swallowing.

When foods are mixed with saliva they form a *bolus*, or ball that is propelled backward via the tongue for swallowing into the *esophagus*, a short tube that is lined with saliva for moisture and protection. A cartilage flap covers the esophagus that prevents the bolus from entering the *trachea* or windpipe.

The esophagus is actually a band of strong muscles that pump and propel food to the stomach. At the end of the esophagus is the cardiac sphincter, a valve that closes the opening once the bolus enters the stomach.

If the cardiac sphincter does not operate properly, then foods and beverages may back up from the stomach and cause acid reflux that may be controlled by a number of factors such as diet, medications, smaller meals, or surgery.

Stomach

Once inside the stomach, stomach enzymes, along with *hydrochloric acid* (a strong acid that digests proteins) and mucous, break down foods and beverages that contain proteins. Muscular contractions then help to convert the bolus into *chyme*, a semifluid of partially digested foods and gastric fluids.

Carbohydrates and fats are fairly undigested in the stomach; they move into the small intestine for additional digestion.

Small Intestine

The small intestine is small in diameter but long in uncoiled length (about 20 to 23 feet in total and about one inch in diameter). It contains three sections: the *duodenum*, *jejunum* and *ileum*. Together they work with the *gallbladder*, *liver*, and *pancreas*—three organs that secrete substances into the small intestine that continue to digest chyme.

The *duodenum* is short; it prepares the absorption of nutrients by mixing chyme from the stomach, digestive fluids from the pancreas, and bile from the liver. The *jejunum* is located in the midsection of the small intestine where the products of nutrient digestion (amino acids, fatty acids, and sugars) are absorbed. The *ileum* mainly absorbs bile acids, vitamin B12, and other remaining nutrients.

The *gallbladder* secretes *bile* (an emulsifier that contains cholesterol) into the small intestine to help digest fats. The *liver* detoxifies metabolites, participates in metabolism, produces biochemicals for digestion, regulates glycogen storage, and synthesizes proteins among many other functions. The liver also produces bile that is stored in the gallbladder. This is why the liver is so vital.

The *pancreas* also secretes substances into the small intestine for digestion. Pancreatic secretions help to neutralize acidic chyme from the stomach and its digestive enzymes help to further digest carbohydrates, fats, and proteins respectively.

The pancreas produces *insulin* and *glucagon*, two important *hormones* essential in carbohydrate metabolism for maintaining blood glucose (sugar). Insulin is secreted by the beta cells of the pancreas to handle elevated blood glucose, while alpha cells of the pancreas secrete glucagon in response to low blood glucose. The pancreas is also a very critical body organ.

Large Intestine

The large intestine is shorter in length (about 5 feet) but larger in diameter (about 3 inches) than the small intestine. It contains the *cecum*, *colon*, and *rectum*.

What is not absorbed by the small intestine moves into the large intestine and blends with water and minerals. There is some vitamin absorption, but essentially the main functions of the large intestine are to hold and help excrete the remains of digested foods and beverages via its strong muscles.

Factors That Affect Healthy Digestion

An intact and fully functional digestive tract provides the framework for healthy digestion and metabolism. Activity level, conditions and diseases, diet, genes, medications, stress, and other factors may affect healthy digestion.

Good vs. Bad Bacteria

Bacteria, *fungi*, and *viruses* are miniscule microbes that reside in the intestines as well as inside the genitalia, mouth, nose, urinary tract, and on the skin. A microbiome is a collection of these microbes that is unique for each individual. It is determined by genetics and lifestyle among other factors.

In the bigger picture, microbiome disruption and/or bacteria imbalances may be associated with conditions or diseases such as colon cancer, diabetes, and obesity. Microbiome bacteria imbalances may also contribute to *inflammatory autoimmune diseases* such as inflammatory bowel disease including Crohn's disease, lupus, and rheumatoid arthritis.

Modifying one's microbiome through environmental and lifestyle changes may provide some insights into these diseases and others and outline courses of action.

Healthy Gut Flora

Since gut bacteria line the intestines, they are involved with the digestion and absorption of foods and beverages. Gut bacteria also help communicate with the body's immune system, influence brain functioning, and produce vitamins that are necessary for life.

It's possible that people with GI conditions and diseases have different compositions of gut bacteria that affect these functions and others. It may also be that a *diversity* of gut bacteria is more important than the presence or absence of specific gut bacteria.

Imbalanced gut bacteria may also be linked with attention-deficit-disorder, anxiety, autism, Alzheimer's disease, cardiovascular disease, and depression. This is because gut bacteria may be able to produce *metabolites*, or small molecules than may make their way to the brain, heart, and other organs and affect their normal functioning.

Improving Gut Flora

Gut flora may improve with a diet that is lower in fats and sugars and higher in certain fibers. By making certain dietary changes, a person may be able to alter their microbiome, improve their immune function, reduce inflammation, and be healthier overall. Drinking more water, managing stress, and incorporating exercise into daily activities may also help support a healthier microbiome.

Healthy gut bacteria may be increased through the addition of *fermented foods* with *probiotics*, live bacteria and yeasts that include certain types of yogurt, kefir (a yogurt-based beverage), miso, pickles, and sauerkraut. Another option is the use of *probiotic supplements* with similar functionality. Probiotic supplements are thought to be safe but they may have side effects and/or trigger allergic reactions.

People with depressed immune function due to chemotherapy or late-stage cancer should be cautioned about taking probiotic supplements since they may be incompatible with treatments.

Digestive Disorders

When a finely tuned digestive system becomes misaligned, a host of GI disorders and systemic issues may arise that may affect a number of other bodily functions.

Digestive disorders from simple stomachaches to more complicated diseases, such as celiac disease or gluten intolerance, may impact this very intricate yet naturally ongoing biological process of digestion. This may be due to bacteria and/or enzyme disorders, stomach acid imbalances, inflammation, and other states.

Symptoms

Common symptoms of GI disorders may include any or many of the following conditions: abdominal pain/syndrome, acid reflux, belching, biliary tract disorders, bloating, constipation, dyspepsia, flatulence (gas), gallbladder disorders, gallstone pancreatitis, gastro-esophageal reflux disease, heartburn, hemorrhoids, indigestion, irritable bowel syndrome, nausea, peptic ulcer disease, vomiting, and more.

Identification

Imaging tests such as abdominal ultrasound, abdominal X-ray, computed tomography (CT) scan, CT angiography, magnetic resonance imaging (MRI), radionuclide scanning, virtual colonoscopy, and upper and lower GI tests may be used to detect GI irregularities.

Upper GI tests may be used to examine the esophagus, stomach, and duodenum and to diagnose esophageal variances, hiatal hernias, obstruction, or narrowing of the upper GI tract, tumors, ulcers, and other anomalies.

Lower GI tests may be used to detect Crohn's disease, colon polyps, diverticular disease, gastroenteritis, strictures or site narrowing and/or obstruction, tumors, ulcerative colitis, and more.

Body awareness may be the first identification of GI disorders and defense. Regular medical examinations may detect underlying symptoms.

Food Allergies, Intolerances, and Sensitivities

An *allergy* is an immune system disorder. A food allergy or *hypersensitivity* is a reaction to a substance in a food or beverage.

An allergic food reaction occurs when a substance in the environment that is known as an allergen prompts an allergic reaction by the human body. Common allergic reactions to foods and beverages may include asthma, eczema, hay fever, hives, and GI reactions.

In contrast, *food intolerance* is hypersensitivity to a non-allergic food or beverage. By and large, food intolerance does not provoke an abnormal response to the proteins in foods and beverages, though some of the symptoms may be similar. These may include aches and pains, bloating, cramping, diarrhea, headaches, heartburn, irritability, nausea, stomach pain, and/or vomiting.

In general, food intolerances are more common than diagnosed food allergies. For example, gluten and lactose intolerance are considered food intolerances, not allergies since they may not be triggered by the immune system nor life-threatening.

In general, the removal of suspected foods and beverages that are connected with food intolerances may be effective for remedying symptoms.

The term *food sensitivity* is sometimes used interchangeably with food intolerance. Food sensitivities imply that there are sensitive reactions to food, rather than intolerance that may be mild, not immediate nor life-threatening.

Food sensitivities may be mainly digestive in nature and may not become evident for sometime after a suspected food or beverage is consumed.

Gluten Intolerance and Sensitivity

Gluten intolerance is the inability of the human body to tolerate the protein gluten. Gluten intolerance is different from a wheat allergy in that it is a severe and sudden response to wheat.

Gluten intolerance is actually due to *gliaden*, a component of gluten that is responsible for the action of bread to rise. Gliaden prompts the autoimmune system to react to the tissues in the small intestine and produce an inflammatory response. The *villi* (small hair-like projections that protrude from the intestinal wall) become flattened and unable to assist nutrient transport and absorption into the bloodstream. This may be detected by biopsies or blood tests.

Many foods and beverages contain gluten that is obvious, hidden, or sometimes unexpected. Gluten may be found in common and ancient grains that include barley, brewer's yeast, bulgur, couscous, kasha, malt (including malt extract, malt flavoring, malt syrup, malt vinegar, malted barley flour and malted milk, or milkshakes), matzo meal, oats, rye, triticale, and wheat and its varieties and derivatives (such as durum, einkorn, emmer, farina, farro, graham, kamut, semolina, spelt, and wheat berries).

Other substances in foods and beverages that may contain gluten include artificial and natural flavorings, hydrolyzed plant or vegetable proteins, and modified food starches that may be found in beer, cold cuts, egg substitutes, frozen yogurt and yogurt drinks, salad dressings, and other foods.

Tolerated grains may include corn, millet, quinoa, rice, sorghum and teff. Amaranth and pure buckwheat may also be tolerated since they are botanically considered as grains. Root and legume starches (such as arrowroot, pea, potato, or soybean) may be used in combination with tolerated grains to replicate the action of wheat-based products.

Celiac Disease

In the larger picture, gluten intolerance is considered a symptom of *celiac disease*, an autoimmune disorder of predisposed people that affects the GI tract. Symptoms of celiac disease may include anemia, diarrhea, fatigue, and/or weight loss. If damage to the small intestine occurs, then lactose intolerance may result.

Celiac disease may lead to deficiencies in vitamins A, D, E and K, folic acid, vitamin B12, calcium, and iron and generate to abdominal bleeding, anemia, and/or osteoporosis.

In comparison, *non-celiac gluten sensitivity (NCGS)* is a susceptibility to gluten in foods, beverages, and ingredients. It is not diagnosed food intolerance. NCGS is characterized by intestinal and other bodily symptoms that are related to the ingestion of foods and beverages with gluten.

By adhering to a gluten-free diet, the small intestine may be able heal and symptoms may subside, but there is no known cure for celiac disease.

Irritable Bowel Syndrome

Irritable bowel syndrome (IBS) is a common functional disorder of the GI tract that may produce abdominal pain, bloating, change in bowel habits, constipation, diarrhea, and/or gas. IBS is often included in the spectrum of gluten-related disorders along with celiac disease, non-celiac gluten sensitivity, and wheat allergy. IBS is unlike *inflammatory bowel disease* in that there is not inflammation, ulcers, or damage to the bowel.

The diagnosis of IBS is based on clinical characteristics. Alterations in intestinal motility, permeability, nutrient absorption, and intestinal microbiota (gut flora) may be indicated. Anorexia, fever, GI bleeding, and/or severe weight loss may signify a more acute situation.

Contributing factors that may lead to IBS may include alterations in brain-gut signaling, changes in the gut microbiome, genetics, impaired gut barrier functions, immune dysfunction, and psychosocial factors.

Trigger foods and beverages, particularly ones that evoke hypersensitivity to food antigens, are also implied as is accelerated colonic transit.

Dietary modifications that address IBS include the reduction of gas-producing foods such as *Fermentable Oligo-*, *Di-* and *Monosaccharides and Polyols*, (referred to as FODMAPs), gluten, and lactose.

Dietary and other approaches to IBS include an elimination diet, high and low-fiber diet, low-fat diet, gluten-free and lactose-free diets, and low-FODMAP diet in addition to decreased caffeine, increased water consumption, regular exercise, and mindfulness training.

Crohn's Disease

Crohn's disease is a chronic inflammatory disease characterized by inflammation of the GI tract. While Crohn's disease may affect any part of the GI tract from the mouth to the anus, it most often affects the small intestine. Crohn's disease may also affect the eyes, joints, and skin.

Compared to *ulcerative colitis* (another inflammatory bowel disease), Crohn's disease may appear in patches, extend through the entire thickness of the bowel wall, and have a high rate of relapse. What makes Crohn's disease different and potentially more serious than irritable bowel syndrome is its chronic inflammation.

Lactose Intolerance, Sensitivity, and Milk Allergy

Lactose intolerance is the inability of the human body to digest, metabolize, and absorb the milk sugar *lactose* that is found in some dairy milk and milk products. There is a higher incidence of lactose intolerance in countries and ethnicities where dairy milk and products are not commonly consumed, such as Africa, Asia, Central American, and the Middle East. Lactose intolerance may also increase with age if there is a reduction or absence of the enzyme *lactase* that is responsible for its breakdown.

Lactase (located in the lining of the small intestine) breaks down lactose into *glucose* and *galactose*, two simple sugars to be metabolized for energy. With insufficient lactase, lactose may collect in the small intestine since it may not be able to pass through the villi into the bloodstream. Instead, lactose may accumulate and be metabolized by intestinal bacteria that may cause fermentation and a range of symptoms. These may include bloating, cramping, diarrhea, or gas.

A heightened reaction to lactose may be detected by a blood sugar test, elimination of dairy products, hydrogen breath test, physical exam, or stool sample.

Lactose sensitivity may not clearly be detected as reactions may be sporadic. *Milk allergy* is an allergic response that involves the immune system to the protein (usually casein or whey) in milk.

Human milk is high in lactose. Buffalo, cow, goat, sheep, and yak milk contain about equal amounts of lactose that is about one-half that of human milk. Some dairy products and butters that are fat-free or reduced in fat tend to have milk solids added, so they may be higher in lactose.

Products with less lactose include some hard cheeses, such as Parmesan, fermented cheeses such as cottage cheese, soft cheeses such as ricotta, and ice cream. Buttermilk, sour cream, and yogurt may contain some lactase that is produced by bacteria during their manufacture.

Food additives with lactose may include lactoserum, margarine, milk solids, modified milk ingredients, and whey that may be found in nondairy foods that include processed breads, meal-replacement products, and some meats.

Lactose drops and tablets may be taken before dairy products are consumed to aid their digestion. But the best strategy is avoidance. Bean, grain, and nut "milks" and some modified dairy-alternative products are available. They should be fortified with the nutrients that dairy products normally provide, especially calcium and vitamins A and D.

Leaky Gut Syndrome

Leaky gut syndrome may be more of a collection of symptoms than a diagnosed medical condition. A diagnosis of "leaky gut" may be difficult to establish due to the complexities of the gut and its immunological implications. Symptoms of "leaky gut syndrome" (as increased intestinal permeability) may appear as bloating, cramps, food sensitivities, gas, and general aches and pains.

Increased intestinal permeability is thought to be a possible cause of leaky gut syndrome. Tight junctions in the gut that control what passes through the small intestine may work improperly and permit substances to leak into the bloodstream. This condition may trigger inflammation and changes in gut flora that may lead to digestive changes and complications.

Some people who have celiac or Crohn's disease may experience leaky gut, but little more is known. The standard American diet that is low in fiber and high in saturated fats and sugars may likely play a role along with chronic stress, heavy alcohol use, and lifestyle. Some people may have a genetic predisposition.

Leaky gut may be associated with other autoimmune diseases and conditions such as acne, allergies, arthritis, asthma, chronic fatigue syndrome, fibromyalgia, lupus, mental illness, multiple sclerosis, obesity, and/or type 1 diabetes, but clinical studies do not demonstrate cause and effect. A nutritious whole foods diet with foods and beverages that help to suppress inflammation and the avoidance of those that promote inflammation may be the most defensive.

FODMAPs

FODMAPs (Fermentable Oligosaccharides, Disaccharides, Monosaccharides and Polyols) are a collection of tiny carbohydrate molecules that are naturally found in some foods in the human diet. FODMAPs may be poorly digested and absorbed by some individuals and may reach the end of the intestine where some gut bacteria reside. These bacteria may feed on FODMAPs and produce hydrogen gas, rather than methane gas that is produced by friendly bacteria.

As a result, some digestive symptoms such as bloating, constipation, diarrhea, distention, gas, and/or stomach pain may result. In particular, FODMAPs tend to be "osmotically active" which means that they may pull water into the intestine and contribute to bloating and diarrhea.

During the digestive process, when carbohydrates (starches and sugars) are broken down into their components, some are considered "short-chain" with only a few sugar molecules linked together. These include *fructose, fructans, galactans, lactose,* and *polyols*.

Fructose is a sugar that is naturally found in some fruits and vegetables and in "added sugars". *Fructans* are found in gluten-containing grains such as barley, rye, and wheat. *Galactans* are present in legumes. *Lactose* is found in dairy products and *polyols* appear in sugar alcohols such as *sorbitol, mannitol,* and *xylitol* and in some fruits and vegetables such as some apples, carrots, corn, pineapple, and plums.

A *low-FODMAP diet* is a dietary approach that may be used by some people who have *functional gastrointestinal disorders (FGID)* or irritable bowel diseases such as Crohn's disease and ulcerative colitis. A low-FODMAP diet plan limits foods, beverages, and other substances that contain foods and beverages with FODMAPs.

How the Low-FODMAP Diet works

By eliminating foods and beverages that are high-FODMAPs and focusing on those that are low-FODMAPs, gastrointestinal symptoms may be reduced or eliminated. The more diligent that a person is in eliminating high-FODMAPs, then the more relief that they may experience.

However, instead of eliminating all high-FODMAPs, it is possible to eliminate one suspected food or beverage and observe any reactions before reintroducing or avoiding that food or beverage. This is the basis of an elimination diet that is often used to detect suspected allergens. An elimination diet may also be used in conjunction with medical tests for fructose, gluten, or lactose intolerance to rule out specific reactions to these substances.

High-FODMAP foods and beverages to exclude or limit include:

Beverages such as beer, fruit juices, high fructose corn syrup, milk, soft drinks with high-fructose corn syrup, and soy milk.

Breads, cakes, and cookies such as breads (including sourdough), bread crumbs, cakes, cookies, and sweet breads that contain rye or wheat.

Cereals such as mixed-grain, muesli, and wheat-based.

Dairy products such as fresh or soft cheeses; frozen yogurt, ice cream, milk from dairy cows, goats, and sheep; sour cream, many yogurts; and whey protein supplements.

Fruits such as fresh apples, apricots, blackberries and boysenberries, cherries, dates, figs, pears, peaches, watermelon, applesauce, and canned fruits.

Flours and grains such as barley, bulgur, chickpea flour*, couscous, durum, kamut, lentil flour*, multigrain flour, pea flour*, rye, semolina, soy flour*, triticale, wheat bran, wheat flour, and wheat germ.
as tolerated

Legumes such as baked beans, canned beans that include chickpeas and kidney beans, lentils and soybeans, and fresh legumes.

Nuts and seeds such as cashews and pistachios.

Pasta and noodles such as those made with mixed grain or wheat flours.

Sweeteners such as fructose, high fructose corn syrup, honey and sugar substitutes such as maltitol, mannitol, sorbitol, and xylitol.

continued on next page

Vegetables such as artichokes, asparagus, beets, broccoli, Brussels sprouts, cabbage, cauliflower, fennel, garlic, mushrooms, okra, onions, leeks and shallots, and peas.

Wheat products such as many breads, biscuits, breakfast cereals, crackers, pancakes, tortillas, and waffles.

- -

In contrast, Low-FODMAP foods and beverages to incorporate include:

Beverages such as mineral or soda water, natural spring and mineral water, and many coffees and teas.

Breads, cookies, and cakes such as corn tortillas and taco shells, plain rice cakes and crackers, and gluten-free products.

Cereals such as corn or rice-based breakfast cereals, cream of buckwheat or rice, oatmeal, and gluten-free products.

Dairy products such as ripened cheeses that include Brie and Camembert, hard cheeses that include Parmesan and Romano, and dairy-free dairy products (lactose-free milk, kefir, and yogurt).

Eggs*

Fats and oils such as butter (without milk solids), ghee, lard, and vegetable oils.

Fish*

Fruits such as bananas, blueberries, cantaloupe and other melons except watermelon, grapefruit, kiwifruit, lemons, limes, mandarins, oranges, passion fruit, raspberries, and strawberries.

Flours, grains, and starches such as arrowroot, buckwheat flour, cornmeal, cornstarch, glutinous rice, ground rice, malt, millet, oat bran, oatmeal, polenta, popcorn, potato flour, quinoa, rice, rice bran, rice flour, sago, sorghum, tapioca, wild rice, and gluten-free products.

Herbs and spices (without sweet fillers)

Meats*

Nuts and seeds such as almonds, cashews, Macadamia, and pine nuts and sesame seeds and their "butters" (without sweeteners).

Pasta and noodles such as glass (mung bean) noodles, pure buckwheat soba noodles, rice noodles, and rice vermicelli.

Poultry*

Sweeteners such as maple syrup, molasses, some artificial sweeteners (other than high-FODMAP), and stevia.

Vegetables such as bok choy, carrots, celery, chives and green onions, cucumbers, eggplant, green beans, kale, leafy green lettuces, parsnips, potatoes, radishes, spinach, squash including zucchini, sweet potatoes, tomatoes, turnips, water chestnuts, and yams, along with alfalfa sprouts, and the rhizome ginger root.

*without added High-FODMAP ingredients

Understanding the Nutrition Facts Label

The *Nutrition Facts Label* found on food products was designed to aid consumers in their food and beverage selections. By checking the Nutrition Facts Label and ingredient list, a person may be able to select foods and beverages with the most nutrients and least amount of excess calories, sugars, fats, sodium, and some additives and preservatives that might be detrimental to health.

Reading and comprehending the Nutrition Facts Label and ingredient list are especially important for people with GI disorders to help avoid potential food and beverage triggers before consumption.

As you review the Nutrition Facts Label, take into account these guidelines.

To Decrease Acidity

- Look for common food acids: ascetic acid (vinegar), citric acid, fumaric acid, lactic acid, malic acid, and tartaric acid.

- Consider the pH value of foods and beverages. Generally citrus fruits and juices (grapefruits, lemons, and oranges) have a low pH. Apples, blueberries, grapes, mangoes, peaches, pineapples, plums and pomegranates also tend to be acidic, as are some black coffee, milk, and sodas.

- Balance acidity with fresh vegetables (that include aloe vera, fennel, parsley, and root vegetables such as potatoes) and other more alkaline foods and substances such as bananas, bulgur wheat, couscous, fish and seafood, ginger, oatmeal, poultry, and rice.

To Decrease Fats and Oils:

- Look for these terms that indicate fats or oils in an ingredient list:

    Cholesterol, fatty acids, hydrogenated or partially hydrogenated oils, lecithin, margarine, monounsaturated fatty acids, polyunsaturated fatty acids, saturated fatty acids, total fat, trans fatty acids, oils (such as canola, corn, olive, peanut, safflower, soybean, sunflower and vegetable oil), omega-3 and 6-fatty acids, solids fats (such as butter, beef fat [tallow], chicken fat, coconut oil, pork fat [lard], shortening, palm oil, and palm kernel oil.

To Decrease or Eliminate Gluten

- Look for the following ingredients that generally indicate a product contains gluten:

  - Barley

  - Brewer's yeast

  - Malt (such as barley malt or malt vinegar); maltodextrin may be safe to consume.

  - Oats (unless certified gluten-free since may cross-contaminate).

  - Rye

  - Wheat and derivatives (such as modified food starch).

- *"Wheat-free"* does not necessarily ensure that a product is gluten-free.

To Decrease or Eliminate Lactose

- Look for the following terms that generally indicate that a product contains the milk sugar lactose:

  - Butter
  - Casein
  - Caseinates
  - Cheese
  - Curds
  - Dried milk powder
  - Dry milk Solids
  - Lactose
  - Lactose monohydrate
  - Milk by-products
  - Nonfat dry milk
  - Nougat
  - Whey

- Avoid products with the term *"may contain milk or milk solids"*.

- Plant-based milk substitutes that are made from almonds, oats, rice, and soy should not contain lactose and may be tolerated. They are sometimes referred to as plant "milks".

- Baking and binding agents, lactate, *lactitol* (a sugar alcohol), lactic acid, lactic acid bacteria (fermented lactic acid in sauerkraut, for example), milk protein and starches, and thickening agents do not tend to contain lactose.

- Lactose may also be present in prescription and over-the-counter medications, including some calcium chews and ones that are used for gas or stomach acid.

To Decrease or Eliminate Wheat

- Look for the following terms that generally indicate a product contains wheat:

  - All-purpose flour, bread made with wheat or white flour, bread crumbs, bread flour, bulgur, cereal extract, couscous, cracker meal, einkorn, emmer (farro), farina, flour, graham, gluten, kamut, malt, malt extract, matzo and matzo meal, noodles, pasta, semolina, spelt, sprouted wheat, tabbouleh, triticale, triticum, wheat berries, wheat bran, wheat germ, wheat germ oil, wheat grass, wheat starch, whole wheat bread, whole wheat flour.

  - Some artificial and natural flavorings, caramel color, dextrin, food starch, gelatinized starch, modified starch, modified food starch, vegetable starch, glucose syrup, hydrolyzed vegetable protein (HVP), maltodextrin, monosodium glutamate (MSG), oats, soy sauce (also shoyu, tamari and teriyaki sauce), surimi, texturized vegetable protein, and vegetable gums may also contain wheat.

- The term "wheat" may appear in parentheses in an ingredient list or a separate "*contains*" statement. According to the Food Allergen Labeling and Consumer Protection Act as one of the top eight allergens, wheat must be clearly identified on a food label. Derivatives of wheat, such as "*modified food starch*" must also be clearly identified.

To Decrease or Eliminate FODMAPs

- Look for the following terms on food labels that generally indicate a product contains FODMAPs:

  - Oligosaccharides and fructans—found in barley, cashews, chamomile tea, dates, dried figs, fennel tea, garlic, inulin (as in chicory root), leeks, legumes, nectarines, onions, oolong tea, pistachios, plums, prunes, rye, shallots, soybeans, watermelon, wheat, and white peaches.

  - Disaccharides (lactose)—found in cream cheese, cottage cheese, ice cream, milk, ricotta, and yogurt.

  - Monosaccharides (fructose)—found in agave, apples, asparagus cherries, high fructose corn syrup, fresh figs, honey, Jerusalem artichokes (sun chokes), mangoes, pears, sugar snap peas, and watermelon.

  - Polyols (sorbitol and mannitol)—found in apples, apricots, blackberries, cauliflower, mushrooms, nectarines, peaches, pears, plums, prunes, snow peas, sweet corn, and watermelon.

To Increase Probiotics

- Look for the following terms that generally indicate a product contains probiotics:

  - Buttermilk
  - Fermented milks
  - Kefir
  - Kim chi
  - Miso
  - Sauerkraut
  - Some juice
  - Some pickles
  - Some soft cheese
  - Some yogurt
  - Soy drinks
  - Tempeh

- Dietary probiotics have various forms and functions, such as *acidophilus* (in yogurt and other fermented foods), *bifidobacterium* (in some dairy products such as some cheeses and yogurt), and *saccharomyces boulardii* (yeast found in some probiotic supplements). It is best to investigate what's right.

To Decrease or Increase Dietary Fiber

- Many foods and ingredients are sources of dietary fiber. Look for the following terms:

  - Foods with *insoluble fibers*: avocados, bananas, cauliflower, celery, grapes, green beans, kiwi fruit, legumes, nuts and seeds, tomatoes, zucchini, and whole grains.

  - Foods with *soluble fibers*: apples, avocados, barley, berries, broccoli, carrots, figs, flax, Jerusalem artichokes, legumes, nuts (especially almonds), oats, onions, pears, plums, psyllium, prunes, and sweet potatoes.

Deciphering Food Additives and Preservatives

Different GI problems may require the avoidance of specific food additives or preservatives. This is especially the case for FODMAPs.

In general for lactose intolerance or sensitivity, avoid additives or preservatives that include "lactose" or "lactose monohydrate".

For gluten sensitivity or intolerance, avoid artificial food colorings, artificial sweeteners, butylated hydroxytoluene (BHT) and butylated hydroxyanisole (BHA), brominated vegetable oil (BVO) and added vegetable gums.

Some food colorings, flavor enhancers, or additives may or may not contain gluten such as caramel color, hydrolyzed plant protein, maltodextrin, maltose, modified food starch, monosodium glutamate (MSG), natural and artificial flavorings, and textured vegetable protein. It's best to check directly with food manufacturers.

Dietary Challenges and Assistance

If there are one or two GI conditions or diseases, then dietary strategies may be straightforward, such as the elimination of gluten or lactose for intolerances. Dietary approaches for multiple GI conditions or diseases may be mindboggling.

The best course of action is to discover what works best for you. Note these step-by-step strategies:

Evaluate Food/Beverage Triggers

When certain foods and/or beverages cause discomfort or pain, see if avoidance produces relief. Maybe their frequency needs to be reduced. By substituting other foods or beverages, symptoms may dissipate. This step takes trial and error.

Eliminate Food Triggers

"Trigger foods", even in tiny amounts, may elicit allergic responses, such as hives, breathing problems, GI symptoms, or even anaphylaxis (a severe allergic reaction that may impair breathing and cause shock).

For example, wheat gluten may instigate intestinal cramping, but people with a wheat allergy may have a severe allergic reaction such as asthma, hives, skin rash, or intense stomach disorders such as diarrhea, vomiting, or at worst anaphylaxis.

An *elimination diet* may be used to exclude suspected food and beverage triggers and identify potential allergic or sensitive foods and beverages. A health care provider or team should closely monitor allergic individuals who undergo an elimination diet because some substances may provoke acute reactions.

Other than an elimination diet, blood and skin tests may also help to identify problematic substances.

Determine which Foods/Beverages to Avoid, Limit, and Include

The goal of a gut-healthy diet is to eliminate certain foods and beverages that are suspected of provoking symptoms; limit others that may be intermittently tolerated, and support remaining foods and beverages for inclusion and well-being. This may vary according to individualized needs so one overall gut-healthy dietary approach may be complicated.

Evaluate Other Factors

Fiber is important for healthy digestion since it serves to push foods through the GI tract, create volume and weight to the feces to make it softer and easier to pass, and provide fullness and satisfaction.

- A fiber-rich diet has been connected to decreased incidences of certain cancers, cardiovascular disease, diabetes, and other chronic conditions and diseases. These disorders may be reduced by the inclusion of fresh fruits and vegetables, legumes, nuts and seeds, and whole grains, if tolerated.

Hydration is essential for fiber to be effective. Water is vital for many bodily functions involved in healthy digestion, including the effective use of fiber. Natural spring and mineral water are best options.

The amount of water that one consumes may lead to constipation or diarrhea. If too little water is consumed, then more salts and water are absorbed from the bowel and the chances of constipation may increase. If too much water is consumed, then this may lead to bloating or acid reflux by flushing the stomach contents into the esophagus.

- Soda and other soft drinks should be avoided since they may add carbonation, excess calories, and sugars. Pure fruit and vegetables juices may still be high in calories and sugars. Caffeinated coffees and teas may stimulate the gut. Some herbal teas might cause some sensitivities since they may cross-react with food allergens. Unsweetened dairy milk alternatives provide protein and vitamin and mineral-rich options.

- Alcoholic beverages should only be used in moderation, if tolerated, since alcohol may impair muscle function and contribute to heartburn and diarrhea, damage the musical lining of the esophagus, increase the risk of esophageal cancer, and impair nutrient absorption.

Processed foods are often higher in calories and some fats, sodium, and sugars that are counter-indicated for gut-healthy eating. When in doubt, select foods and beverages that are in their most natural states and farm-raised, grass-fed, in-season, and organic as much as possible.

Probiotics may be used to support a well-chosen gut-healthy meal plan.

Supplements may have their place in a gut-healthy diet, but a well-formulated food and beverage protocol should be constructed first and then any gaps identified and addressed.

Create a Personalized Plan for Optimal Gut Health

By taking the aforementioned strategies into account a person may be able to create a list of foods and beverages to USE, LIMIT, and AVOID for optimal gut health. With this list, foods and beverages to USE may be divided into meals and snacks. Try to include protein, healthy carbohydrates, and fats at each meal or mini-meal for optimum nutrition and satisfaction.

Journal Foods, Beverages, Exercise, Mindfulness, and Reactions

Journal writing and on-line tracking programs provide opportunities to tag certain foods and beverages, track exercise, program mindfulness, and chart physical and emotional responses. This accounting may be useful for noting which strategies work and which others may need revising.

Plan a Gut-Healthy Food Pantry

Since there is a wide array of GI conditions, an all-encompassing list of gut-health foods and beverages may not be as pinpointed as required. Instead, refer to each of the conditions to learn which foods and beverages to stock or exclude.

Cook Gut-Healthy Foods

One of the most important considerations for gut-healthy cooking is the avoidance of cross-contamination in food and beverage preparation, cooking, and clean up. Even the tiniest amounts of questionable substances may precipitate allergic or sensitivity reactions in prone individuals.

Keep preparation areas sanitized, separate trigger foods and beverages, store foods and beverages separately from non-sanctioned items, and cleanse thoroughly.

Smart cooking techniques that decrease or preserve nutrients without additional calories should be used. These include boiling, broiling, grilling, poaching, steaming, and stir-frying.

Enjoy Stress-Free Eating

Make mealtime as enjoyable as possible by practicing mindfulness and enjoying the companionship of others. For independent living, focus on slowing down, enjoying each mouthful or swallow, placing silverware down between bites, and thinking pleasant thoughts.

Eat Gut-Healthy On-the-Go

Eating and drinking gut-healthy foods and beverages may seem challenging at home; however, gut-healthy dining may be especially difficult when eating out or traveling.

Many restaurant menus are available online which makes reviewing and evaluating menus easier. If questions arise, diners may contact restaurants directly and inquire about specific ingredients and preparations.

Be proactive and inform servers about desirable/undesirable foods and beverages. When in doubt, do not order or share questionable dishes. By ordering plain foods that are simply prepared, some sensitive food triggers may be alleviated. Still, even simple protein foods may be marinated or seasoned with ingredients that precipitate adverse gut reactions.

In general, people with diagnosed allergies, intolerances, or sensitivities should limit or avoid certain restaurants where trigger substances are prominent. A "chef card" may be carried that states food and beverage restrictions. Farm-to-table menus with farm-raised, grass-fed, in-season, organic foods, and beverages may be preferred.

Other Lifestyle Choices

Practice Mindfulness

Mindfulness is the ability to focus the mind on a certain moment and accepting the significances. Mindfulness is both a preventive and therapeutic technique that helps a person to achieve a mental state where bodily sensations, feelings, and thoughts are fairly synchronized. Some people might think of mindfulness as meditation while others might view it as "seizing the moment".

Mindfulness might take backstage to the frantic pace that modern life dictates. For those with GI issues, mindfulness might be "just what the doctor ordered" for calming an over-sensitive GI tract.

The use of mindfulness to handle emotions and stresses that may directly or indirectly affect the gut has been demonstrated in patient studies. Poor gut health has also been implicated in some neurological and neuropsychiatric disorders. By taking the time to slow down, practicing deep breathing and engaging in some calming self-talk, along with a gut-healthy personalized treatment plan, some GI symptoms may be alleviated.

Keep Active

Daily activities and exercise are important for healthy lifestyles that promote mental and physical wellbeing and gut health.

Exercise helps to attain and maintain a healthy weight, enhance nutrient uptake and usage, improve circulation, strengthen the heart and lungs, and support digestion. About 30 minutes of daily exercise is recommended daily.

Regular exercise may also contribute to regular bowel habits since it stimulates the intestinal muscles to contract and push digested substances out of the large intestine through peristalsis and influence normal bowel contraction.

Seeking Additional Help

Chronic gut-related symptoms such as abdominal pain, bloody stool, excessive constipation, diarrhea, distention, gas, and/or sudden weight gain or loss may prompt immediate need for consultation by a health care provider. One that specializes in functional medicine may not only help treat the symptoms but may also try to evaluate the causes and any underlying deficiencies, excesses, or imbalances.

Some examinations and tests might be warranted that include blood chemistry analysis, Elimination Diet, food sensitivity testing, hair mineral analysis, saliva, stool and urine specimen analysis, and/or neurotransmitter profile. Not all of these procedures are considered valid or definitive on their own. They should be viewed comprehensibly for an integrative care approach.

The services of a *Registered Dietitian/Nutritionist (RDN)* may be helpful within the realm of an integrated health care team for devising an individualized gut-healthy diet plan that integrates medications and supplements, if necessary. Make sure that the RDN is a certified provider through the Academy of Nutrition and Dietetics.

Make a Gut-Healthy Lifestyle Work for You

Some people are very motivated to change their diet and lifestyle on their own while others may require major incentives and support. There are both short- and longer-term benefits for undertaking a gut-healthy approach to diet and lifestyle.

For some people, the short-term relief from distressing gastrointestinal symptoms may be encouraging. For others, the hope for longer-term protection from potentially debilitating chronic conditions and diseases may be inspiring. Even if followed to a limited extent, gut-healthy eating and drinking may offer a nutritious approach to foods and beverages, diet, and well-being.

Gut Healthy Recipes

The following pages include more than 85 healthy and easy-to-prepare recipes that may work for you. Take note of your specific condition, whether it is a food intolerance or sensitivity, irritable bowel, leaky gut, or other digestive disorder, and select those recipes with ingredients that are best tolerated. Make modifications, as necessary, that allow these recipes to fit your particular needs.

These recipes were collected with the various "gut" conditions in mind, and given that different foods and beverages work (or don't work) for each condition, you will need to take control of your particular situation to find what works best for you. If your condition persists, seek professional guidance for clarification and a specialized dietary plan.

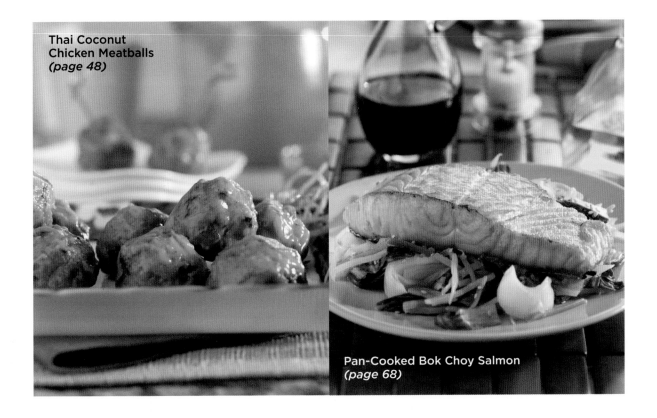

Thai Coconut
Chicken Meatballs
(page 48)

Pan-Cooked Bok Choy Salmon
(page 68)

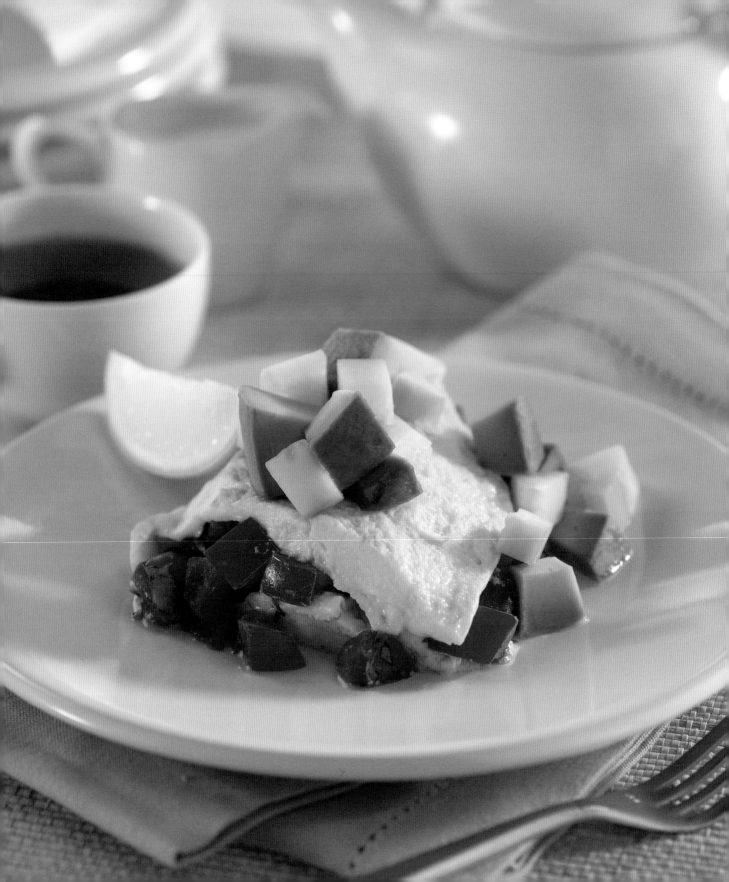

BREAKFAST & BRUNCH

California Omelet with Avocado

MAKES 2 SERVINGS

1 plum tomato, chopped

2 to 4 tablespoons chopped fresh cilantro

¼ teaspoon salt

6 eggs

¼ cup almond milk

1 ripe medium avocado, diced

1 small cucumber, chopped

1 lemon, quartered

1 Preheat oven to 200°F. Combine tomato, cilantro and salt in small bowl; set aside.

2 Whisk eggs and milk in medium bowl until well blended.

3 Heat small nonstick ovenproof skillet over medium heat; coat with nonstick cooking spray. Pour half of egg mixture into skillet; cook 2 minutes or until eggs begin to set. Lift edge of omelet to allow uncooked portion to flow underneath. Cook 3 minutes or until set.

4 Spoon half of tomato mixture over half of omelet. Loosen omelet with spatula and fold in half. Slide omelet onto serving plate and keep warm. Repeat for second omelet. Top with avocado and cucumber. Garnish with lemon.

Super Oatmeal

MAKES 5 TO 6 SERVINGS

2 cups water

2¾ cups old-fashioned oats

¼ cup finely diced dried figs

¼ cup lightly packed dark brown sugar

⅓ to ½ cup sliced almonds, toasted*

¼ cup flaxseeds

½ teaspoon salt

½ teaspoon ground cinnamon

2 cups almond milk

*To toast almonds, spread in single layer on baking sheet. Bake in preheated 350°F oven 8 to 10 minutes or until golden brown, stirring frequently.

1 Bring water to a boil over high heat in large saucepan. Stir in oats, figs, brown sugar, almonds, flaxseeds, salt and cinnamon. Immediately add milk. Stir well.

2 Reduce heat to medium-high. Cook and stir 5 to 7 minutes or until oatmeal is thick and creamy. Spoon into individual bowls.

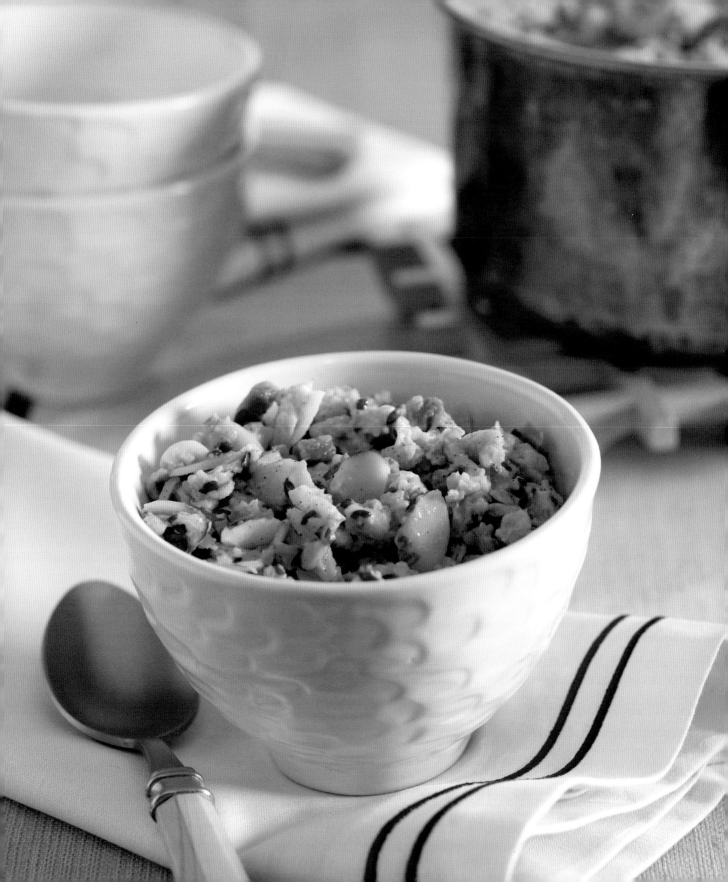

Scrambled Egg & Zucchini Pie

MAKES 2 SERVINGS

2 **eggs**

1 **tablespoon grated Parmesan or Cheddar cheese (optional)**

¼ **teaspoon salt**

1 **teaspoon olive oil**

1 **small zucchini, diced**

1 Preheat oven to 350°F.

2 Whisk eggs in small bowl; stir in cheese, if desired, and salt.

3 Heat oil in small nonstick ovenproof skillet over medium-high heat. Add zucchini; cook and stir 2 to 3 minutes or until crisp-tender.

4 Reduce heat to low; stir egg mixture into skillet with zucchini. Cook without stirring 4 to 5 minutes or until eggs begin to set around edge.

5 Transfer skillet to oven and bake 5 minutes or until eggs are set. Cut into wedges to serve.

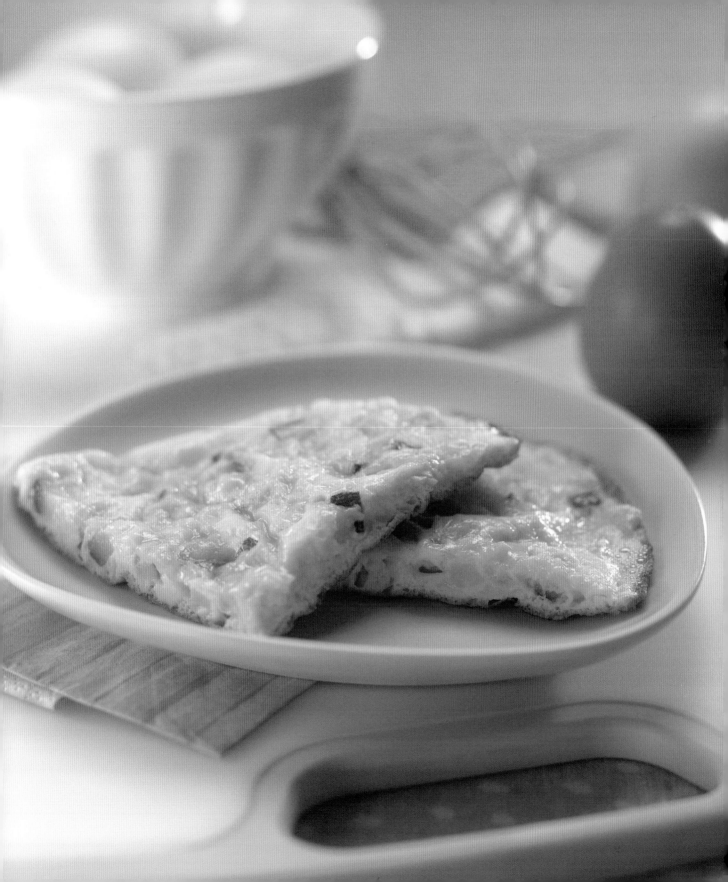

Hash Brown Frittata

MAKES 2 SERVINGS

- ¾ **cup coarsely chopped cherry tomatoes**
- ½ **cup refrigerated hash brown potatoes**
- ¼ **teaspoon salt, divided (optional)**
- ¼ **teaspoon black pepper, divided**
- 4 **eggs**
- ⅛ **teaspoon red pepper flakes**
- ¼ **cup salsa (optional)**

1 Preheat broiler. Coat large nonstick ovenproof skillet with nonstick cooking spray. Add tomatoes. Cook over medium heat 5 minutes or until tomatoes are pulpy, stirring frequently. Add potatoes; press into tomato mixture. Cook over medium heat 5 minutes or until potatoes begin to turn golden. Sprinkle with ⅛ teaspoon salt, if desired, and ⅛ teaspoon pepper.

2 Combine remaining salt, if desired, and pepper, eggs and red pepper flakes in small bowl. Pour into skillet, coating potato mixture. Cook over medium heat until egg mixture is set, turning skillet as needed to cook egg mixture completely.

3 Place skillet in broiler 4 or 5 inches from heat 30 seconds or until egg is set. Cut frittata into wedges. Serve with salsa, if desired.

NOTE

Refrigerated hash brown potatoes are usually available in the produce or egg section of the supermarket.

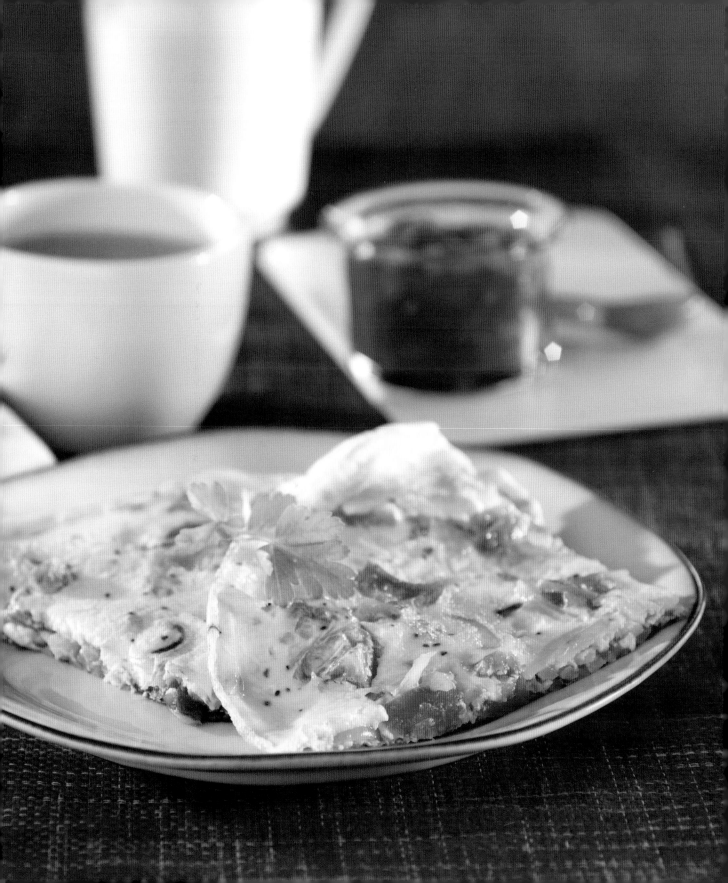

Scrambled Egg Pile Ups

MAKES 1 SERVING

2 **eggs**

2 **tablespoons almond milk**

Salt and black pepper

¼ **cup diced orange bell pepper**

1 **green onion (green part only), finely chopped**

¼ **cup grape tomatoes, quartered (about 6 tomatoes)**

⅓ **cup (about 1½ ounces) shredded Cheddar cheese (optional)**

1 **to 2 tablespoons plain nonfat Greek yogurt (optional)**

1 Preheat waffle maker to medium; coat with nonstick cooking spray.

2 Whisk eggs and milk in small bowl. Season lightly with salt and black pepper. Working quickly, pour egg mixture onto waffle maker, sprinkle with bell pepper, green onion and tomatoes. Close; cook 2 minutes or until puffed.

3 Remove "waffle" to plate; top with cheese and yogurt, if desired. Serve immediately.

TIP

To remove from waffle maker, place a plate over the egg and flip the egg onto the plate. Or, use the tip of a fork to gently release egg from waffle maker, then slide a wide spatula under to gently remove.

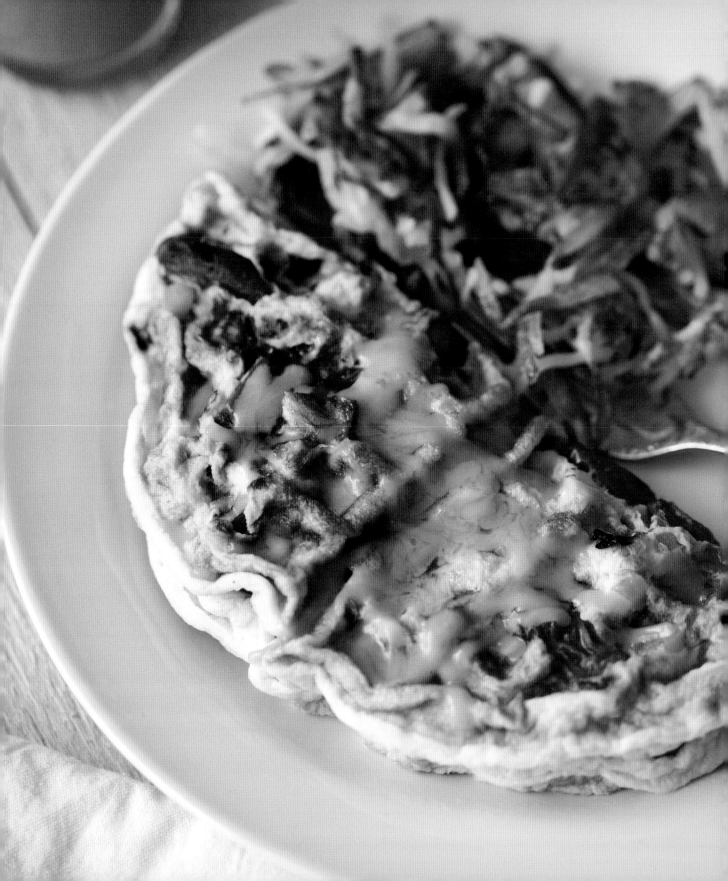

Vegetable Quinoa Frittata

MAKES 6 SERVINGS

1 tablespoon olive oil

1 cup small broccoli florets

¾ cup finely chopped red bell pepper

½ teaspoon garlic powder

1¼ teaspoons kosher salt

Black pepper

1½ cups cooked quinoa

¼ cup sun-dried tomatoes (packed in oil), chopped

8 eggs, lightly beaten

¼ cup grated Parmesan cheese (optional)

1 Preheat oven to 400°F.

2 Heat oil in large ovenproof nonstick skillet over medium-high heat. Add broccoli; cook and stir 4 minutes, Add bell pepper; cook and stir 2 minutes. Add garlic powder, salt and black pepper; cook 30 seconds, stirring constantly. Stir in quinoa and sun-dried tomatoes.

3 Gently stir in eggs; cook until softly scrambled. Sprinkle with cheese, if desired.

4 Bake about 7 minutes or until eggs are set. Let stand 5 minutes before cutting into wedges.

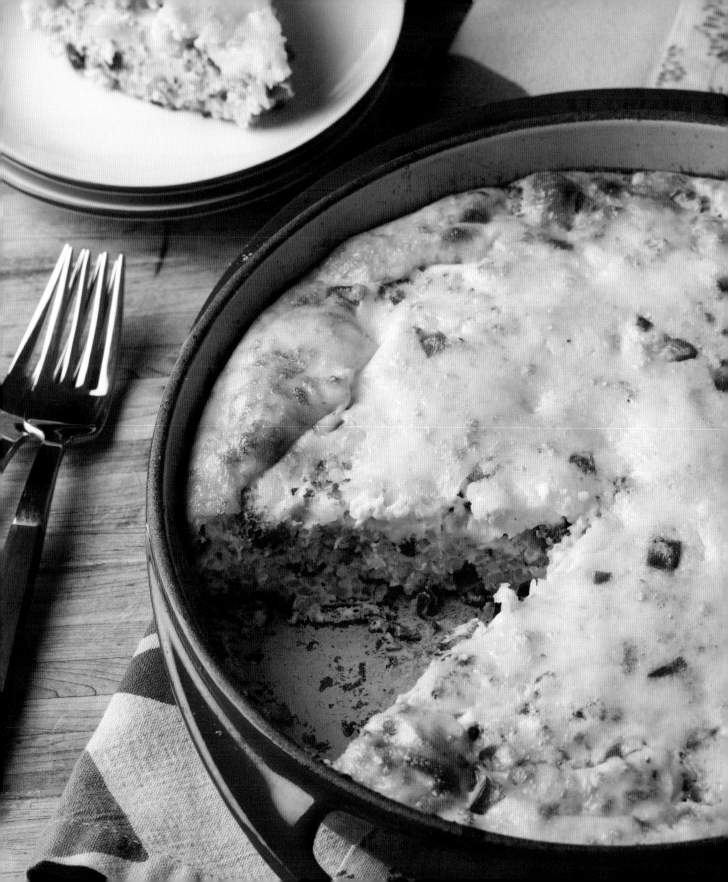

Sizzling Rice Flour Crêpes

MAKES 4 TO 6 SERVINGS

CRÊPES

- 1 cup rice flour
- ½ teaspoon salt
- ½ teaspoon sugar
- ½ teaspoon turmeric
- 1 cup unsweetened coconut milk
- ½ to ¾ cup water
- ½ cup vegetable oil

FILLING

- 1 bunch green onions (green parts only), chopped
- 1 cup chopped cooked chicken *or* 1 cup small raw shrimp, peeled *or* 1 cup cubed tofu
- 2 cups bean sprouts
  Lettuce, fresh cilantro and fresh mint

DIPPING SAUCE (OPTIONAL)

- ⅔ cup water
- ¼ cup gluten-free fish sauce
- 1 tablespoon sugar
  Juice of 1 lime
- 1 serrano or other hot pepper, minced
- 1 to 2 tablespoons shredded carrot

1 Combine rice flour, salt, sugar and turmeric in medium bowl. Gradually whisk in coconut milk and ½ cup water until batter is thickness of heavy cream. Let batter rest at least 10 minutes. Add additional water as needed to thin batter.

2 Heat 9- or 10-inch nonstick skillet over medium heat. Add 3 teaspoons oil to skillet. Add choice of ¼ cup filling to skillet (about 1 tablespoon green onion, plus 3 tablespoons chicken, shrimp, tofu or a combination). Cook and stir 2 to 4 minutes or until onions are softened and shrimp is pink and opaque, if using. Pour about ½ cup batter over filling mixture. Immediately swirl to coat bottom of pan with batter; allow some batter to go up side of pan.

3 In 30 seconds or when sizzling sound stops, add bean sprouts to 1 side of crêpe. Cover pan and cook 3 minutes or until sprouts wilt and center of crêpe appears cooked. Edges should be browned and crisp.

4 Fold crêpe in half with spatula and transfer to plate. Repeat with remaining batter and fillings.

5 For Dipping Sauce, if desired, combine ⅔ cup water, fish sauce, sugar and lime juice in small bowl. Stir until sugar dissolves. Stir in pepper; top with carrot.

6 Serve crêpes with lettuce, herbs and Dipping Sauce, if desired. Traditionally, crêpes are eaten by wrapping bite-size portions in lettuce with herbs and dipping each bite in sauce.

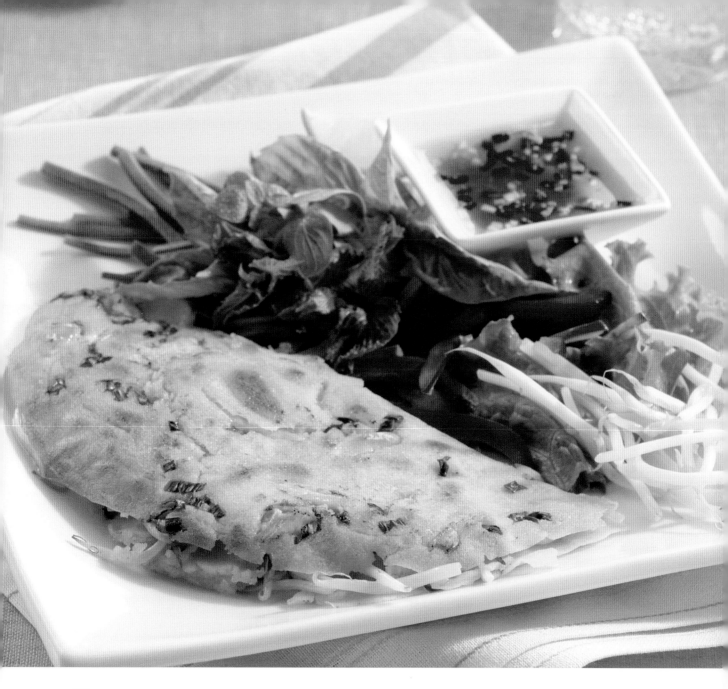

TIP

Sizzling Crêpes (Banh Xeo, pronounced bahn SAY-oh) are a popular
Vietnamese street snack. The word "Xeo" in Vietnamese mimics the sound
the batter makes as it sizzles in the pan. The filling can be almost anything
you wish. Try using leftover pork, beef, vegetables or whatever you have on
hand. Part of the experience is choosing which fresh herbs to add to each
portion of crêpe before wrapping it in a lettuce leaf and dipping it in sauce.
Banh Xeo are a truly hands-on eating experience!

Superfood Breakfast Porridge

MAKES 4 SERVINGS

¾ cup steel-cut oats

¼ cup uncooked quinoa, rinsed and drained

2 tablespoons dried cranberries

2 tablespoons raisins

3 tablespoons ground flaxseeds

2 tablespoons chia seeds

1 teaspoon olive oil

¼ teaspoon salt

¼ teaspoon ground cinnamon

2½ cups almond milk, plus additional for serving

1½ cups water

Maple syrup (optional)

¼ cup sliced almonds, toasted* (optional)

To toast almonds, cook and stir in small skillet over medium heat 1 to 2 minutes or until nuts are lightly browned.

SLOW COOKER DIRECTIONS

1 Combine oats, quinoa, cranberries, raisins, flaxseeds, chia seeds, oil, salt and cinnamon in heatproof bowl that fits inside a slow cooker. Stir in 2½ cups milk until blended.

2 Place bowl in slow cooker. Pour enough water around sides to come up halfway around bowl.

3 Cover; cook on LOW 8 hours.

4 Carefully remove bowl from slow cooker. Stir in additional milk. Top with maple syrup and almonds, if desired.

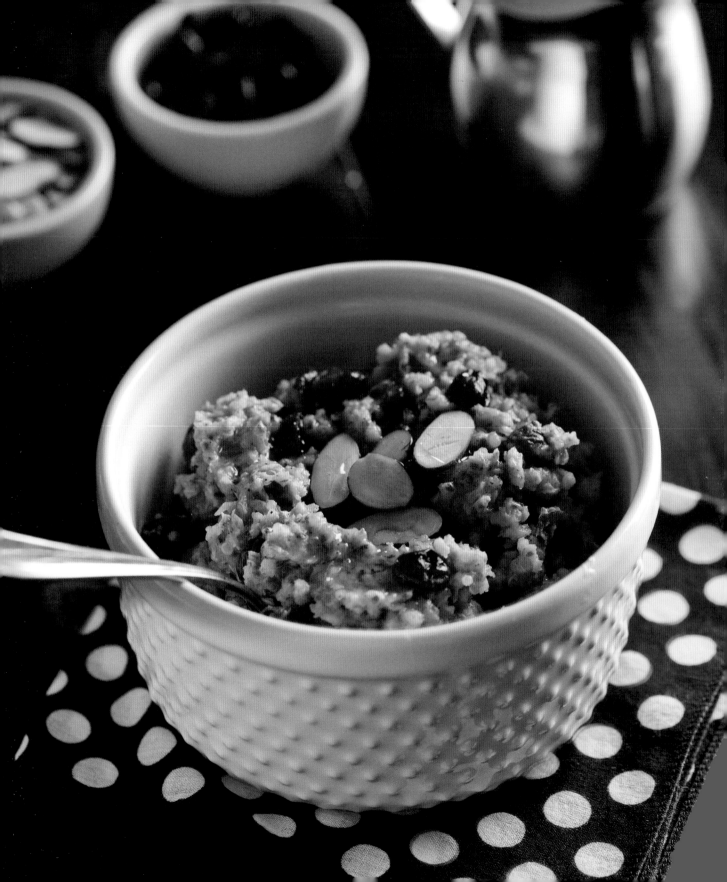

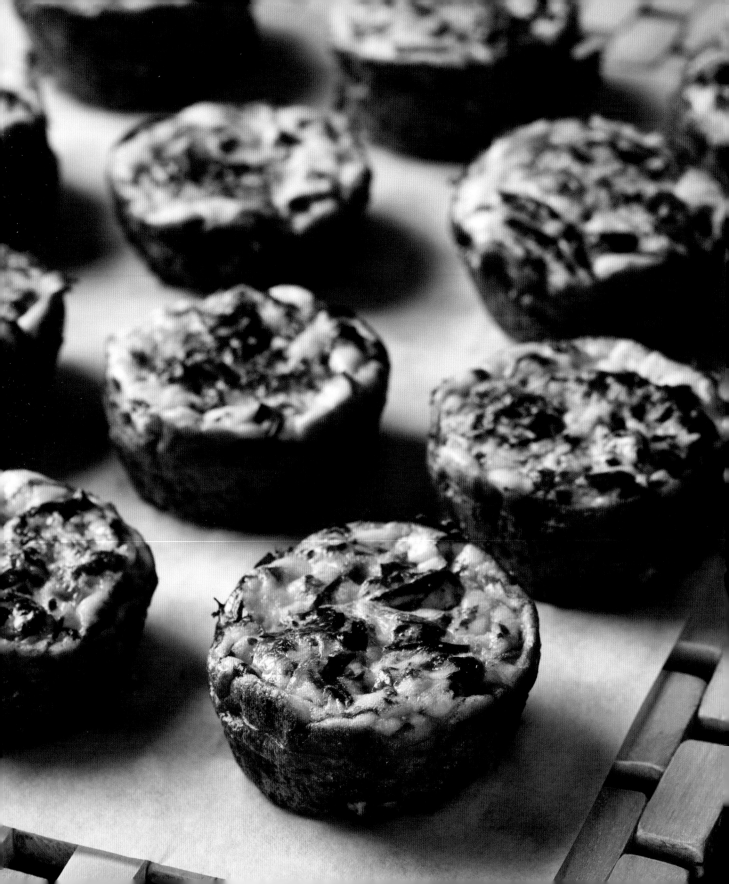

STARTERS & APPETIZERS

Mini Spinach Frittatas

MAKES 12 MINI FRITTATAS (4 TO 6 SERVINGS)

8 eggs

¼ cup plain nonfat Greek yogurt

1 package (10 ounces) frozen chopped spinach, thawed and squeezed dry

¼ cup (2 ounces) shredded white Cheddar cheese

¼ cup grated Parmesan cheese

¾ teaspoon salt

⅛ teaspoon black pepper

⅛ teaspoon ground red pepper

Dash ground nutmeg

1 tablespoon olive oil

1 Preheat oven to 350°F. Spray 12 standard (2½-inch) muffin cups with nonstick cooking spray.

2 Whisk eggs and yogurt in large bowl. Stir in spinach, Cheddar and Parmesan cheeses, salt, black pepper, red pepper and nutmeg until blended. Divide mixture evenly among prepared muffin cups.

3 Bake 20 to 25 minutes or until eggs are puffed and firm and no longer shiny. Cool in pan 2 minutes. Loosen bottom and sides with small spatula or knife; remove to wire rack. Serve warm, cold or at room temperature.

Vegetable-Topped Hummus

MAKES 8 SERVINGS

1 can (about 15 ounces) chickpeas, rinsed and drained

2 tablespoons tahini

2 tablespoons lemon juice

½ teaspoon garlic powder

¾ teaspoon salt

1 tomato, finely chopped

2 green onions (green parts only), finely chopped

2 tablespoons chopped fresh parsley

Oat crackers or fresh vegetable slices (optional)

1 Combine chickpeas, tahini, lemon juice, garlic powder and salt in food processor or blender; process until smooth.

2 Combine tomato, green onions and parsley in small bowl; gently toss to combine.

3 Spoon hummus into serving bowl; top with tomato mixture. Serve with crackers or vegetable slices, if desired.

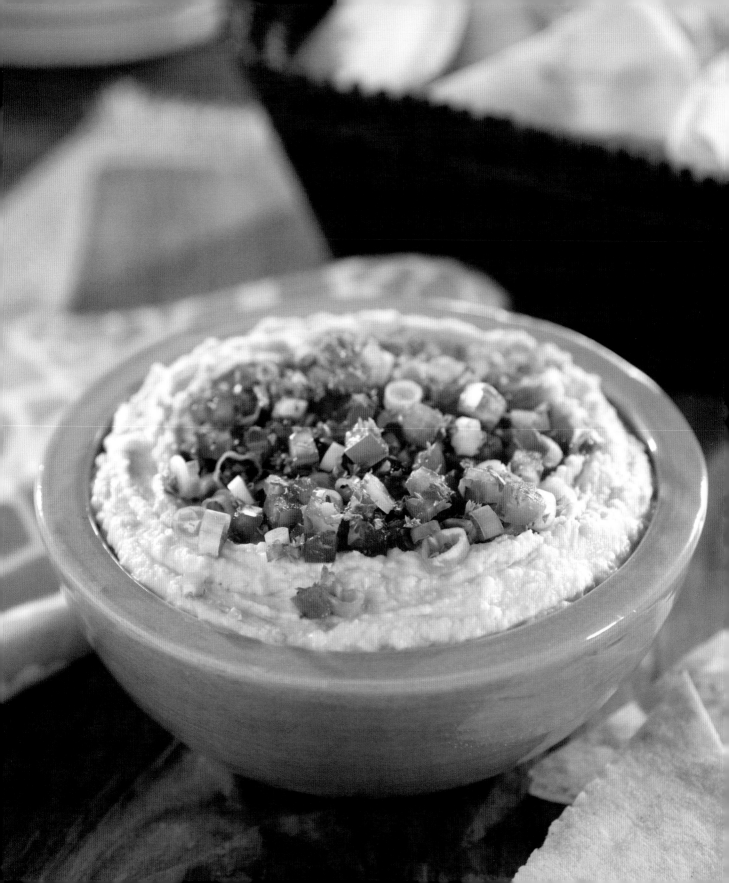

Guacamole

MAKES 2 CUPS

- 2 **large ripe avocados**
- 2 **teaspoons fresh lime juice**
- ¼ **cup finely chopped red onion (optional)**
- 2 **tablespoons chopped fresh cilantro**
- ½ **jalapeño pepper,* finely chopped**
- ½ **teaspoon salt**

Jalapeño peppers can sting and irritate the skin, so wear rubber gloves when handling peppers and do not touch your eyes.

1 Place avocados in large bowl. Sprinkle with lime juice; toss to coat. Mash to desired consistency with fork or potato masher.

2 Add onion, if desired, cilantro, jalapeño pepper and salt; stir gently until well blended.

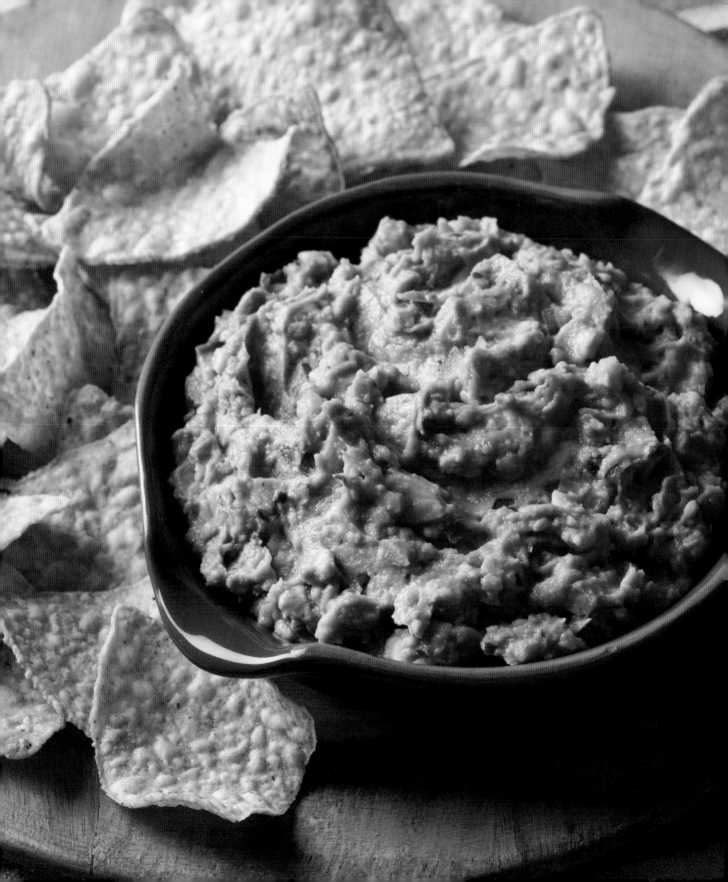

Thai Coconut Chicken Meatballs

MAKES 4 TO 5 SERVINGS

- 1 pound ground chicken
- 2 green onions (green parts only), chopped
- ½ teaspoon garlic powder
- 2 teaspoons dark sesame oil
- 2 teaspoons mirin
- 1 teaspoon fish sauce
- 1 tablespoon canola oil
- ½ cup unsweetened canned coconut milk
- ¼ cup chicken broth
- 1 teaspoon packed brown sugar
- 1 teaspoon Thai red curry paste
- 2 teaspoons lime juice
- 2 tablespoons water
- 1 tablespoon cornstarch

SLOW COOKER DIRECTIONS

1 Combine chicken, green onions, garlic powder, sesame oil, mirin and fish sauce in large bowl. Shape mixture into 1½-inch meatballs.

2 Heat canola oil in large skillet over medium-high heat. Working in batches, brown meatballs on all sides. Transfer to 4½-quart slow cooker. Add coconut milk, broth, brown sugar and curry paste. Cover; cook on HIGH 3½ to 4 hours. Stir in lime juice.

3 Stir water into cornstarch in small bowl until smooth. Whisk into sauce in slow cooker. Cook, uncovered, on HIGH 10 to 15 minutes or until sauce is slightly thickened.

TIP

Meatballs that are of equal sizes will cook at the same rate and be done at the same time. To ensure your meatballs are the same size, pat seasoned ground meat into an even rectangle and then slice into even rows and columns. Roll each portion into a smooth ball.

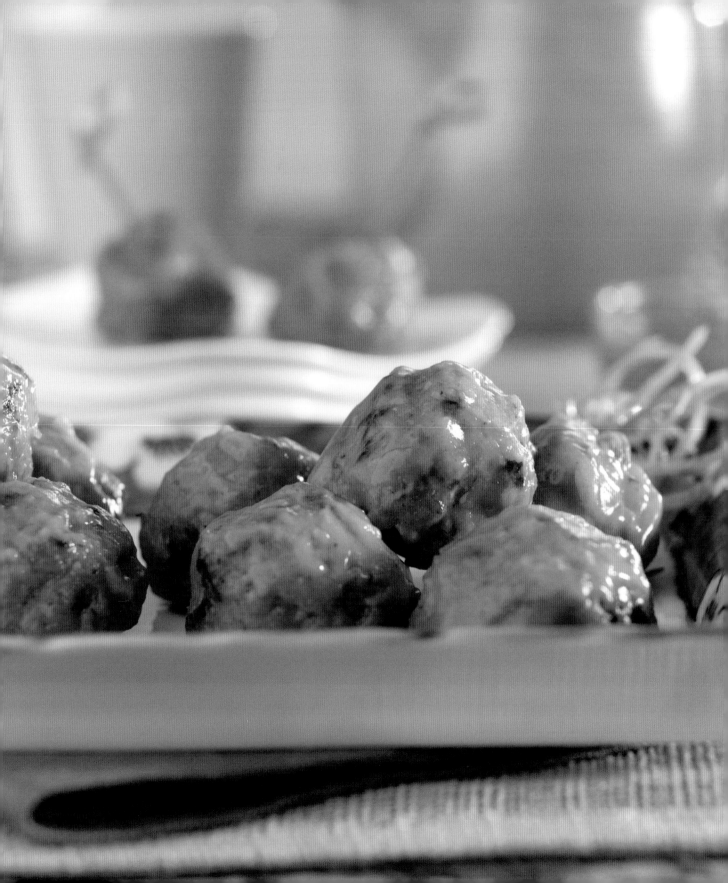

Quick & Easy Hummus

MAKES 4 SERVINGS

- **1 can (about 15 ounces) chickpeas, rinsed and drained**
- **2 tablespoons torn fresh mint leaves (optional)**
- **2 tablespoons olive oil**
- **2 tablespoons lemon juice**
- **2 teaspoons dark sesame oil**
- **½ teaspoon garlic powder**
- **½ teaspoon salt**
- **⅛ teaspoon ground red pepper *or* ¼ teaspoon hot pepper sauce**

With motor running, add all ingredients to food processor. Cover; process until hummus is well combined and is desired consistency (the longer the hummus is processed the smoother the texture).

SERVING SUGGESTION

Serve with vegetable dippers.

TIP

Leftover hummus may be covered and refrigerated up to 1 week.

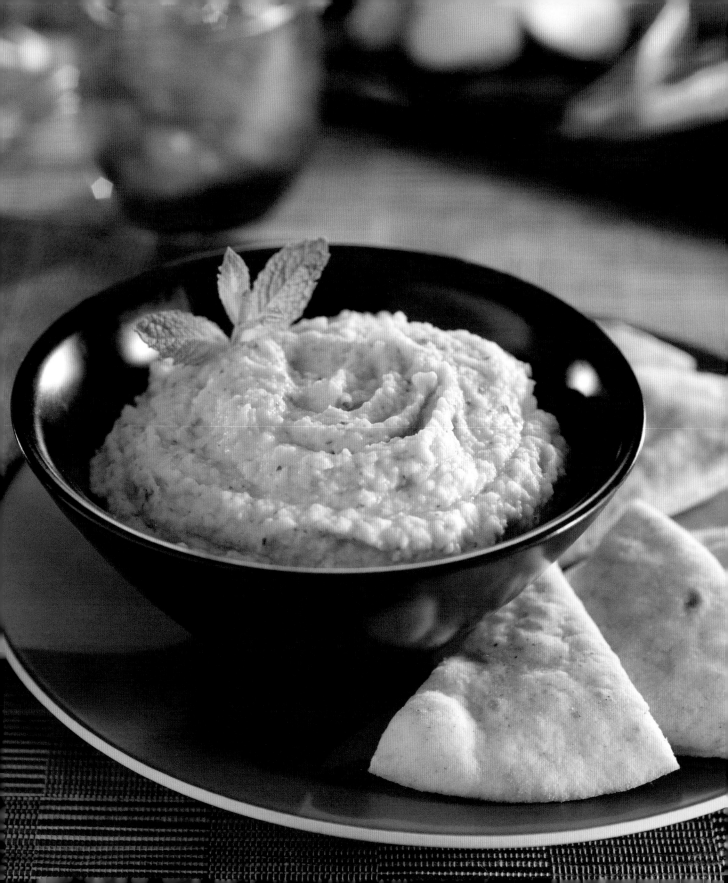

Avocado Smash

MAKES ¾ CUP

1 ripe medium
   avocado

1 tablespoon lime
   juice

¼ cup plain nonfat
   Greek yogurt

1 teaspoon Dijon
   mustard

¼ teaspoon salt

   Chopped fresh
   chives (optional)

Roughly mash avocado with fork in shallow bowl. Stir in remaining ingredients; sprinkle with chives. Serve immediately.

TIP

This dip is great with raw veggies, such as cucumber slices, celery sticks or red bell pepper strips.

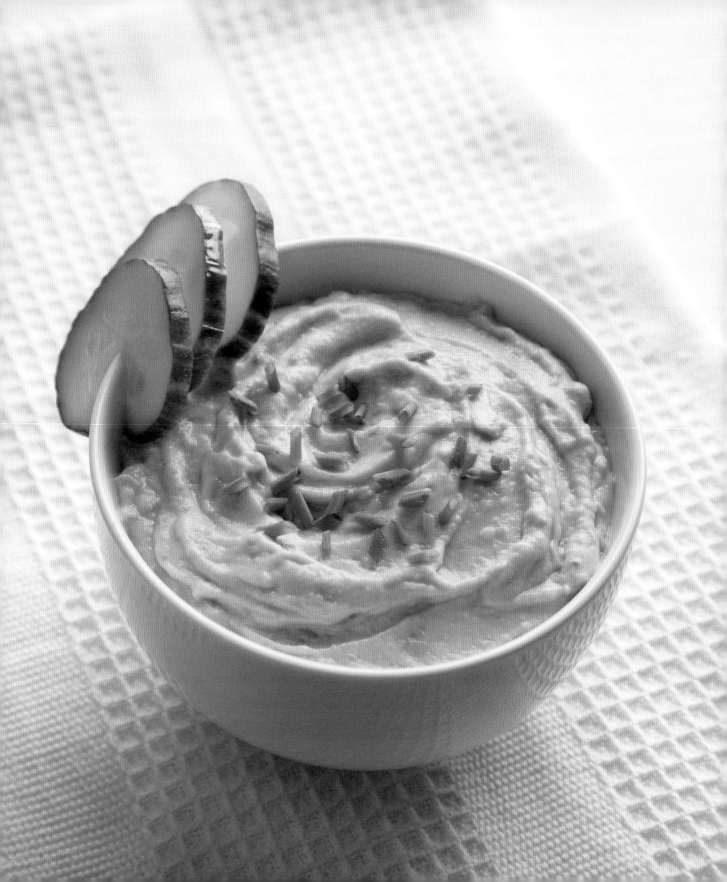

Beef and Lettuce Bundles

MAKES 8 APPETIZER SERVINGS

1 pound ground beef

½ cup green onions (green parts only), finely chopped

⅔ cup chopped water chestnuts

½ cup chopped red bell pepper

1 tablespoon soy sauce

1 tablespoon seasoned rice vinegar

2 tablespoons chopped fresh cilantro

½ teaspoon garlic powder

1 or 2 heads leaf lettuce, separated into leaves (discard outer leaves)

1 Brown beef in large skillet over medium-high heat 6 to 8 minutes, stirring to break up meat. Drain fat. Add green onions; cook until tender. Stir in water chestnuts, bell pepper, soy sauce and vinegar. Cook, stirring occasionally, until bell pepper is crisp-tender and most of liquid has evaporated.

2 Stir in cilantro and garlic powder. Spoon ground beef mixture onto lettuce leaves. Wrap lettuce leaves around beef mixture to make bundles.

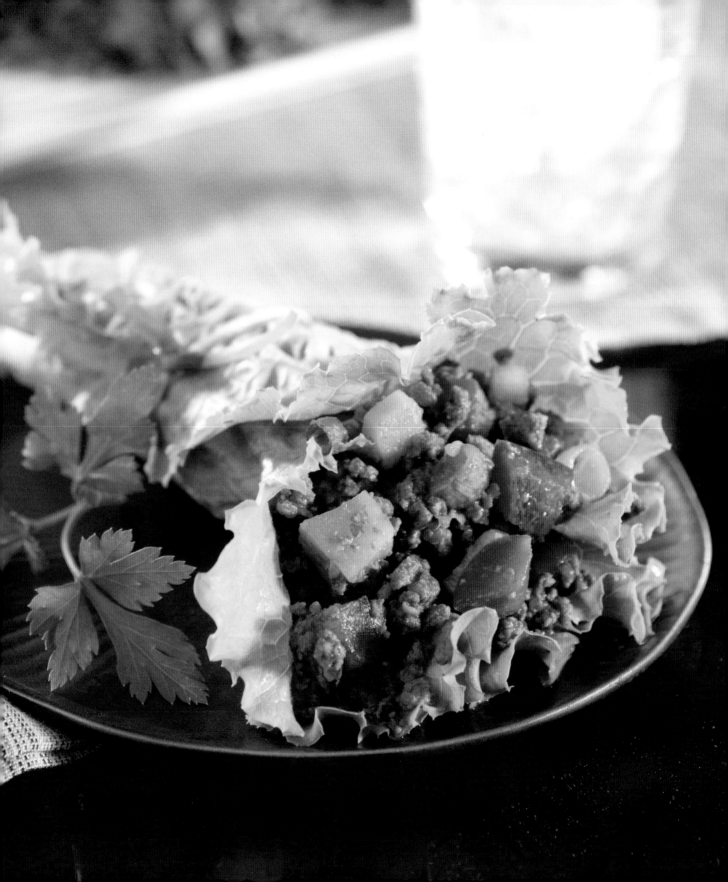

Roasted Eggplant Hummus

MAKES 2 CUPS (ABOUT 16 SERVINGS)

1 **large eggplant**

1 **can (about 15 ounces) chickpeas, rinsed and drained**

½ **teaspoon garlic powder**

3 **tablespoons fresh lemon juice**

2 **tablespoons olive oil**

¾ **teaspoon salt**

¼ **teaspoon ground red pepper**

¼ **cup loosely packed fresh parsley, plus additional for garnish**

Assorted vegetable sticks and/ or gluten-free crackers

1 Preheat oven to 400°F. Cut eggplant in half lengthwise. Place cut side down on baking sheet. Roast 35 to 40 minutes or until tender. Cool completely. Peel eggplant and remove seeds. Reserve pulp.

2 Combine chickpeas and garlic powder food processor; process until finely ground. Add eggplant, lemon juice, oil, salt and ground red pepper; process until smooth. Add ¼ cup parsley; pulse until combined.

3 Serve with assorted vegetable sticks and/or gluten-free crackers. Garnish with additional parsley.

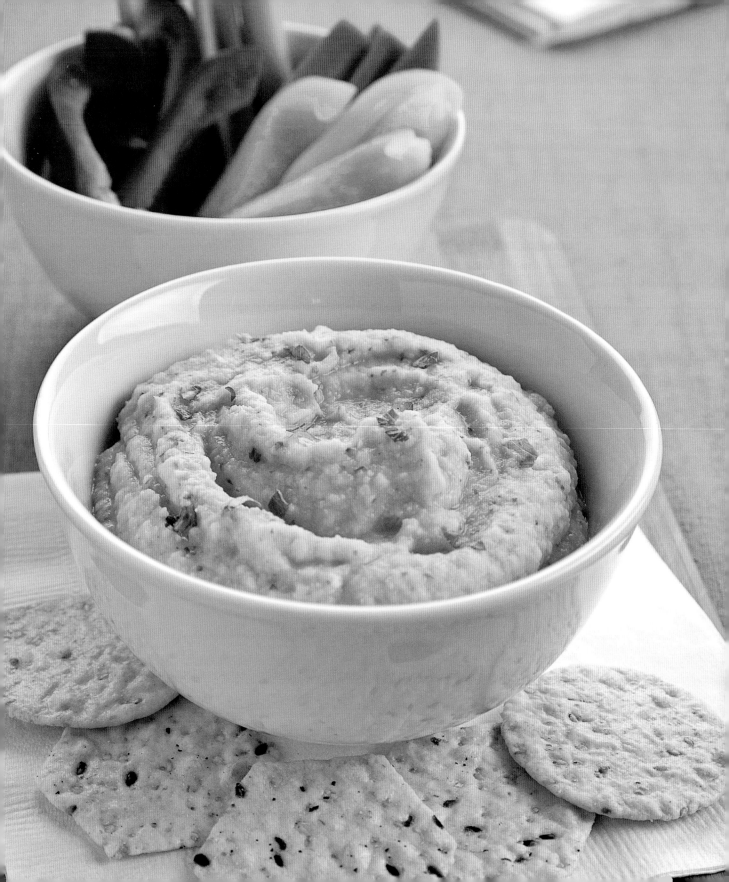

Broiled Shrimp Kabobs

MAKES 4 SERVINGS

2 tablespoons olive oil

2 tablespoons lemon juice

½ teaspoon garlic powder

½ teaspoon salt

½ teaspoon dried oregano

⅛ teaspoon ground red pepper

½ pound medium shrimp, peeled

1 red bell pepper, cut into squares

1 medium zucchini, cut into ½-inch slices

1 Preheat broiler. Whisk together oil, lemon juice, garlic powder, salt, oregano and ground red pepper in medium bowl. Add shrimp, bell pepper and zucchini; stir until well coated.

2 Alternately thread shrimp, bell pepper and zucchini onto skewers.* Place on rack of broiler pan. Broil 4 inches from heat 2 minutes per side or until shrimp turn pink and opaque.

If using wooden skewers, soak in water 20 to 30 minutes before threading.

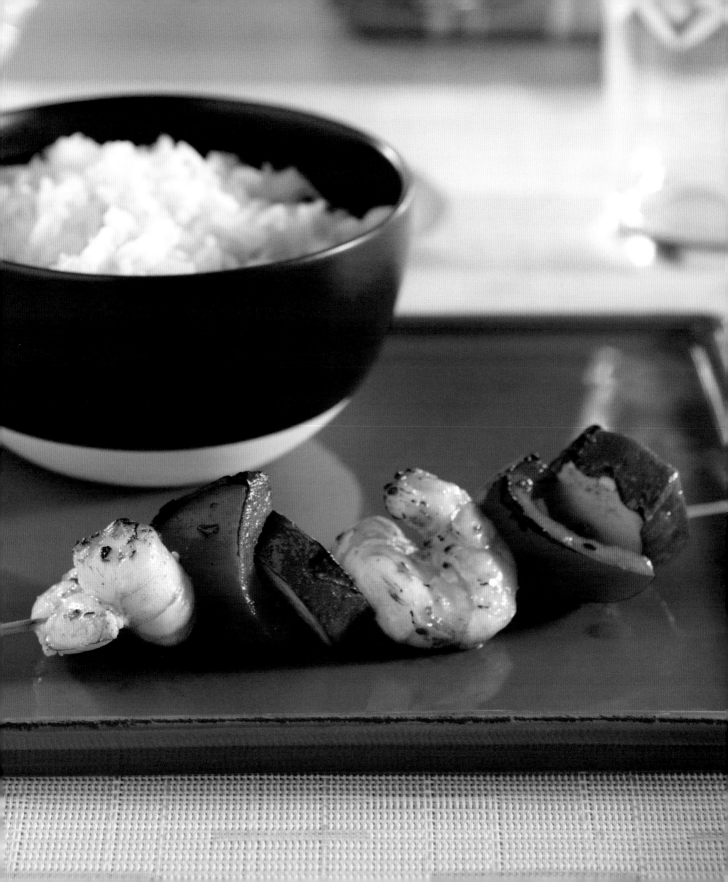

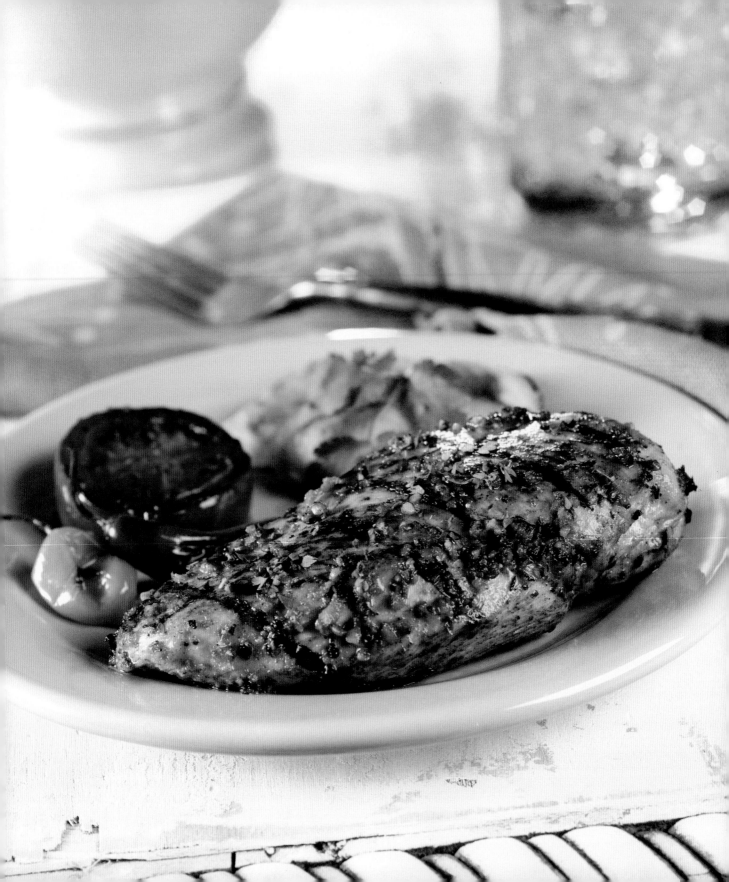

LUNCHES & DINNERS

Grilled Chicken Adobo

MAKES 6 SERVINGS

¼ **teaspoon onion powder**

⅓ **cup lime juice**

1 **clove garlic, coarsely chopped**

1 **teaspoon ground cumin**

1 **teaspoon dried oregano**

½ **teaspoon dried thyme**

¼ **teaspoon ground red pepper**

6 **boneless skinless chicken breasts (about ¼ pound each)**

3 **tablespoons chopped fresh cilantro (optional)**

1 Combine onion powder, lime juice and garlic in large resealable food storage bag. Add cumin, oregano, thyme and ground red pepper; knead bag until blended. Place chicken in bag; press out air and seal. Turn to coat chicken with marinade. Refrigerate 30 minutes or up to 4 hours, turning occasionally.

2 Spray grill grid with nonstick cooking spray. Prepare grill for direct cooking. Remove chicken from marinade; discard marinade. Place chicken on grid. Grill 5 to 7 minutes on each side over medium heat or until chicken is no longer pink in center. Transfer to clean serving platter and garnish with cilantro, if desired.

Lamb Chops with Mustard Sauce

MAKES 4 SERVINGS

1 teaspoon dried thyme

½ teaspoon salt

¼ teaspoon black pepper

4 lamb loin chops (about 6 ounces each)

2 tablespoons canola or vegetable oil

2 tablespoons finely chopped shallots or sweet onion

¼ cup beef or chicken broth

2 tablespoons Worcestershire sauce

1½ tablespoons Dijon mustard

Sprigs fresh thyme (optional)

1 Sprinkle dried thyme, salt and pepper over lamb. Heat oil in large skillet over medium heat. Add chops; cook 4 minutes per side. Remove chops from skillet; set aside.

2 Add shallots to skillet; cook 3 minutes, stirring occasionally. Reduce heat to medium-low. Add broth, Worcestershire sauce and mustard; simmer 5 minutes or until sauce thickens slightly, stirring occasionally. Return chops to skillet; cook 2 minutes for medium rare, turning once. Transfer to serving plates; garnish with fresh thyme.

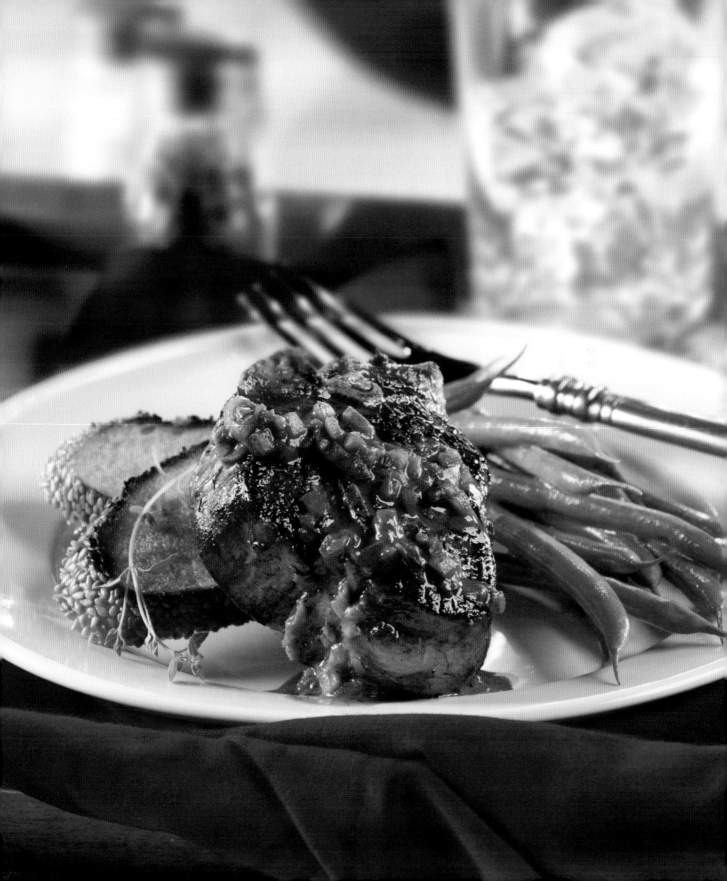

Szechuan Tuna Steaks

MAKES 4 SERVINGS

4 tuna steaks
(6 ounces each),
cut 1 inch thick

¼ cup dry sherry or
sake

¼ cup soy sauce

1 tablespoon dark
sesame oil

1 teaspoon hot chili oil
or ¼ teaspoon red
pepper flakes

½ teaspoon garlic
powder

3 tablespoons
chopped fresh
cilantro (optional)

1 Place tuna in single layer in large shallow glass dish. Combine sherry, soy sauce, sesame oil, hot chili oil and garlic powder in small bowl. Reserve ¼ cup soy sauce mixture at room temperature. Pour remaining soy sauce mixture over tuna. Cover; marinate in refrigerator 40 minutes, turning once.

2 Spray grill grid with nonstick cooking spray. Prepare grill for direct cooking.

3 Drain tuna, discarding marinade. Grill tuna, uncovered, over medium-hot coals 6 minutes or until tuna is seared, but still feels somewhat soft in center,* turning halfway through grilling time. Transfer tuna to cutting board. Cut each tuna steak into thin slices; fan out slices onto serving plates. Drizzle tuna slices with reserved soy sauce mixture; garnish with cilantro.

Tuna becomes dry and tough if overcooked. Cook to medium doneness for best results.

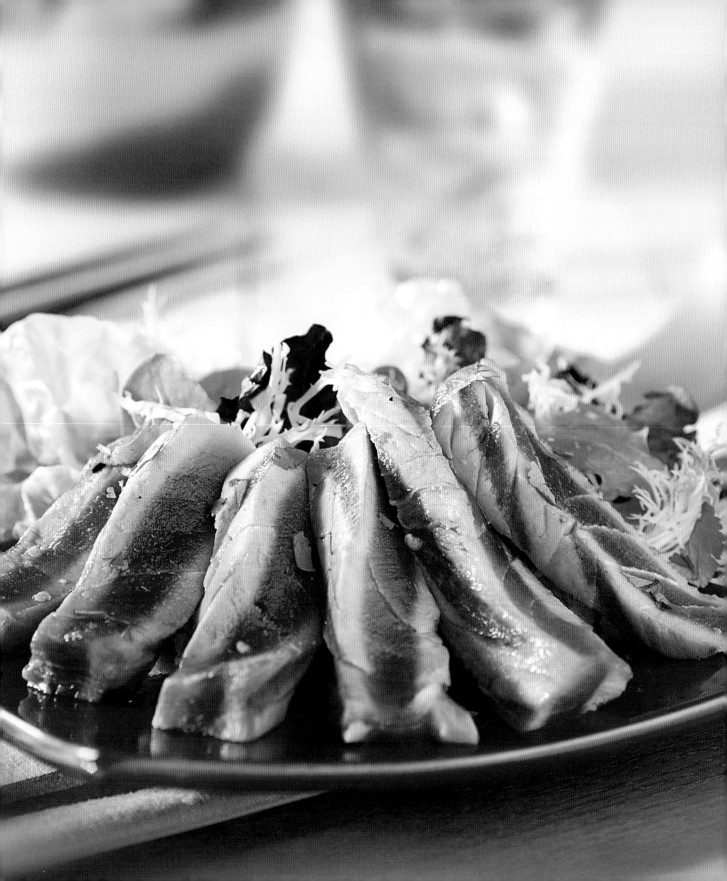

Speedy Salmon Patties

MAKES 3 SERVINGS

1 can (12 ounces) pink salmon, undrained

1 egg, lightly beaten

¼ cup minced green onions (green parts only)

1 tablespoon chopped fresh dill

½ garlic powder

½ cup rice flour

1½ teaspoons baking powder

1 Drain salmon, reserving 2 tablespoons liquid. Place salmon in medium bowl; break apart with fork. Add reserved liquid, egg, green onions, dill and garlic powder; mix well.

2 Combine rice flour and baking powder in small bowl. Add to salmon mixture; mix well. Shape into 6 patties.

3 Spray large heavy skillet with nonstick cooking spray; heat over medium-high heat.

4 Add salmon patties; cook on both sides until golden brown, turning once. Remove using slotted spoon; drain on paper towels. Serve immediately.

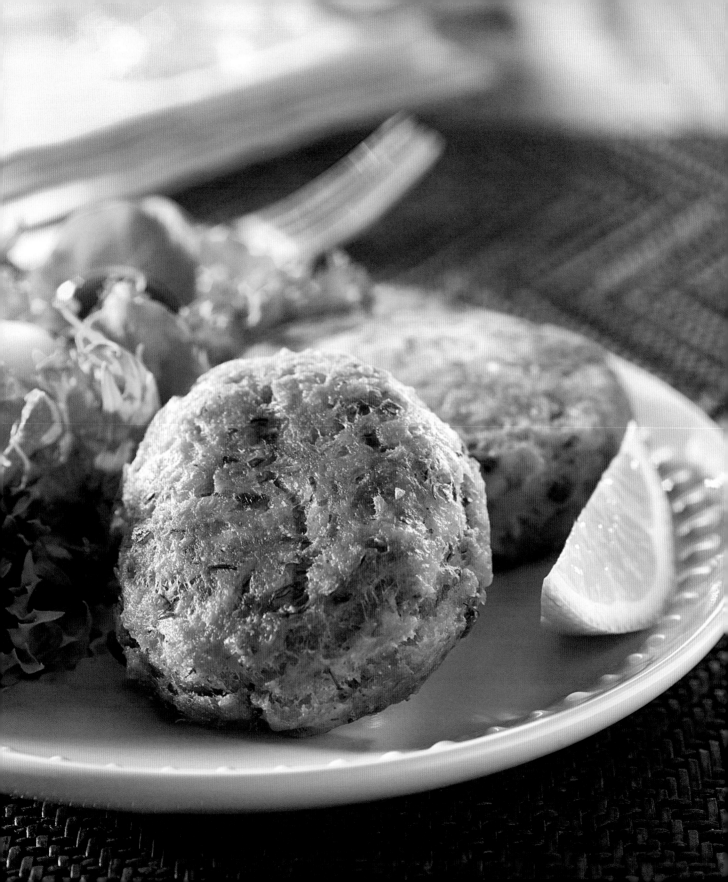

Pan-Cooked Bok Choy Salmon

MAKES 2 SERVINGS

- 1 pound bok choy or napa cabbage, chopped
- 1 cup broccoli slaw mix
- 2 tablespoons olive oil, divided
- 2 salmon fillets (4 to 6 ounces each)
- ¼ teaspoon salt
- ½ teaspoon black pepper
- 1 teaspoon sesame seeds

1 Combine bok choy and broccoli slaw mix in colander; rinse and drain well.

2 Heat 1 tablespoon oil in large nonstick skillet over medium heat. Sprinkle salmon with salt and pepper. Add salmon to skillet; cook about 3 minutes per side. Remove salmon from skillet.

3 Add remaining 1 tablespoon oil and sesame seeds to skillet; stir to toast sesame seeds. Add bok choy mixture; cook and stir 3 to 4 minutes.

4 Return salmon to skillet. Reduce heat to low; cover and cook about 4 minutes or until salmon begins to flake when tested with fork. Season with additional salt and pepper, if desired.

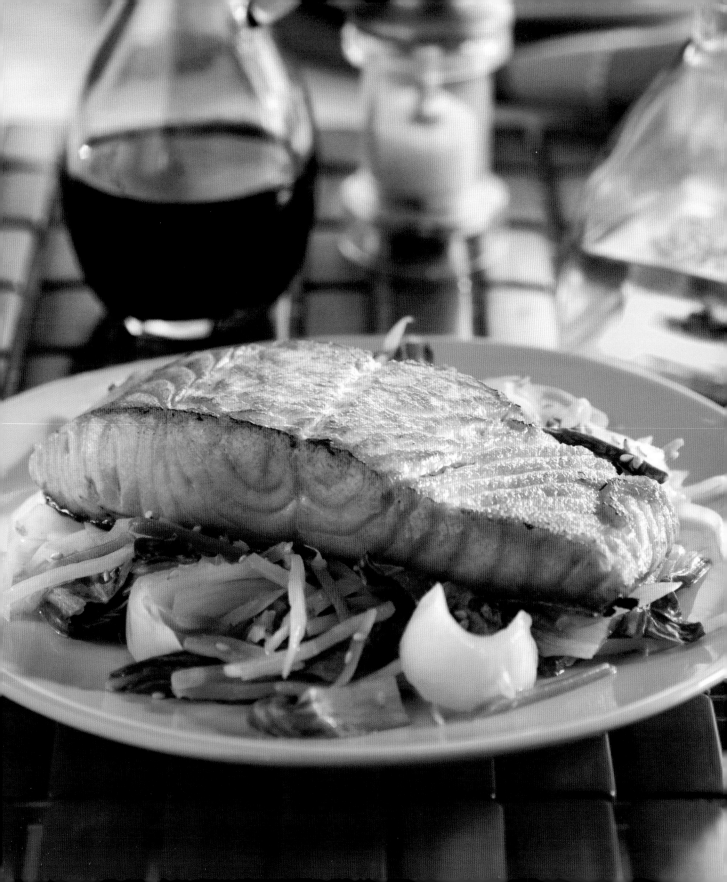

Tilapia with Spinach and Feta

MAKES 2 SERVINGS

1 teaspoon olive oil

4 cups baby spinach

2 skinless tilapia fillets or other mild white fish (4 ounces each)

½ teaspoon garlic powder

¼ teaspoon black pepper

2 ounces reduced-fat feta cheese, cut into 2 (3-inch) pieces

1 Preheat oven to 350°F. Spray baking sheet with nonstick cooking spray.

2 Heat oil in medium skillet over medium-low heat. Add spinach; cook just until wilted, stirring occasionally.

3 Arrange tilapia on prepared baking sheet; sprinkle with garlic powder and pepper. Place one piece of cheese on each fillet; top with spinach mixture.

4 Fold one end of each fillet up and over filling; secure with toothpick. Repeat with opposite end of each fillet.

5 Bake 20 minutes or until fish begins to flake when tested with fork.

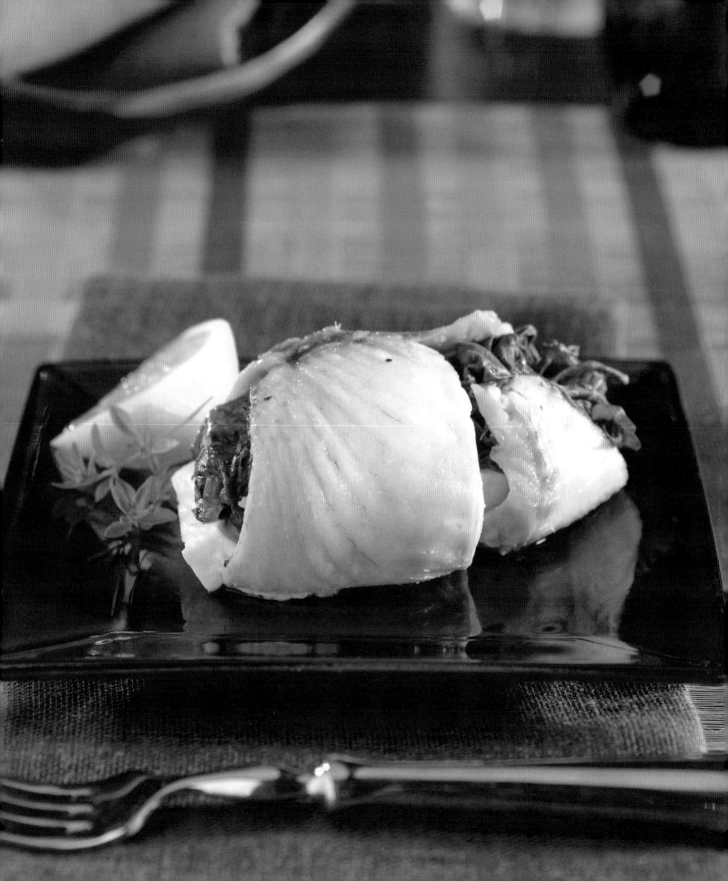

Shrimp and Tomato Salad

MAKES 4 SERVINGS

8 ounces cooked medium shrimp

1 cup cherry tomatoes, halved (or whole small yellow pear tomatoes)

¼ cup chopped or thinly sliced fresh basil leaves

1 tablespoon olive oil

1 tablespoon white wine vinegar

¼ teaspoon freshly ground black pepper

8 large Boston lettuce leaves

½ cup crumbled reduced-fat feta cheese (optional)

Combine shrimp, tomatoes, basil, oil, vinegar and pepper in medium bowl; mix well. Serve over lettuce and top with cheese, if desired.

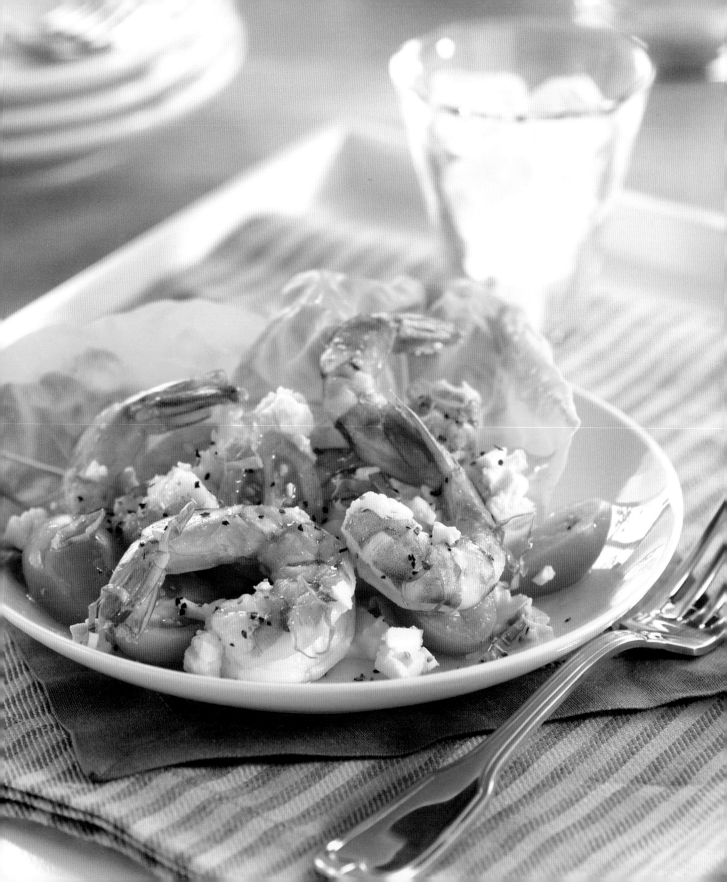

Sesame Peanut Spaghetti Squash

MAKES 4 SERVINGS

1 spaghetti squash (3 pounds)

⅓ cup sesame seeds

⅓ cup vegetable broth

2 tablespoons reduced-sodium soy sauce

1½ teaspoons sugar

2 teaspoons sesame oil

1 teaspoon cornstarch

1 teaspoon red pepper flakes

1 tablespoon vegetable oil

2 medium carrots, julienned

1 large red bell pepper, seeded and thinly sliced

¼ cup fresh snow peas, cut diagonally in half

½ cup coarsely chopped unsalted peanuts (optional)

⅓ cup minced fresh cilantro

1 Preheat oven to 350°F. Spray 13×9-inch baking dish with nonstick cooking spray. Cut squash in half lengthwise. Remove and discard seeds. Place squash, cut side down, in prepared dish. Bake 45 minutes to 1 hour or until tender.

2 Using oven mitts to hold squash, remove spaghetti-like strands with fork. Place strands in large bowl; cover and keep warm.

3 Heat wok or large skillet over medium-high heat. Add sesame seeds; cook and stir 45 seconds or until golden brown. Transfer to blender; add broth, soy sauce, sugar, sesame oil, cornstarch and red pepper flakes. Blend until mixture is coarsely puréed.

4 Heat oil in wok or large skillet over medium-high heat 1 minute. Add carrots; stir-fry 1 minute. Add bell pepper; stir-fry 2 minutes or until vegetables are crisp-tender. Add snow peas; stir-fry 1 minute. Stir sesame seed mixture; add to wok. Cook and stir 1 minute or until sauce is thickened.

5 Serve sauce over spaghetti squash; top with peanuts, if desired, and cilantro.

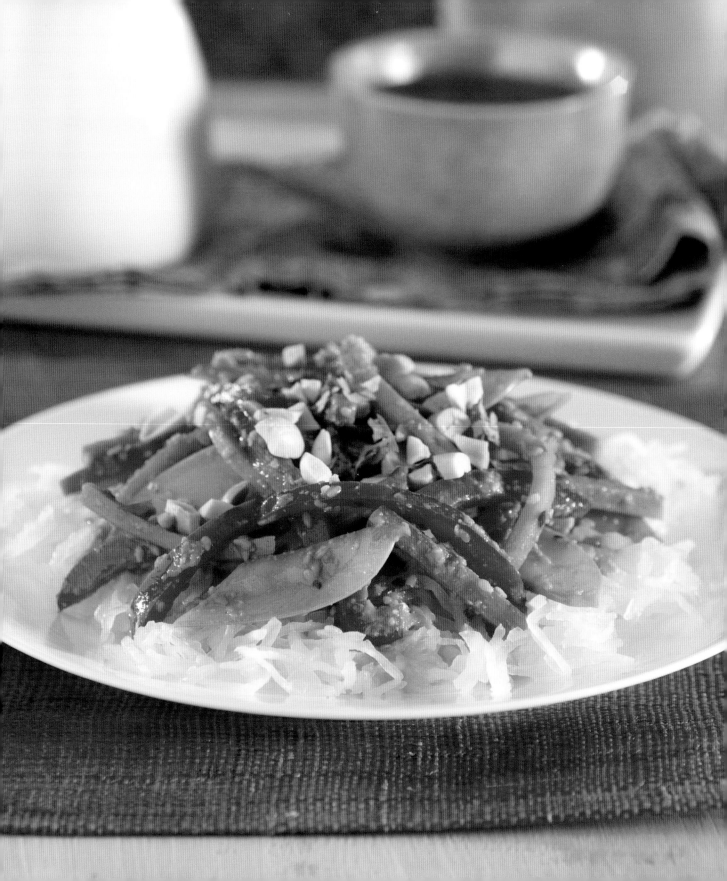

Lemon-Baked Fish with Cajun Buttery Topping

MAKES 4 SERVINGS

3 **medium lemons, divided**

4 **tilapia fillets (about 1 pound total) rinsed and patted dry**

½ **teaspoon dried thyme**

¼ **teaspoon salt**

¼ **teaspoon black pepper**

1 **tablespoon butter**

1 **tablespoon hot pepper sauce (optional)**

2 **tablespoons chopped fresh parsley, divided**

1 Preheat oven to 400°F. Line baking sheet with foil. Slice 2 lemons into 8 rounds total. Arrange lemon rounds in 4 rows (2 slices each). Place 1 fillet on top of each row. (The lemons act as a "bed" for each fillet.)

2 Combine thyme, salt and pepper in small bowl; sprinkle evenly over fillets. Bake 10 to 12 minutes or until fillets are opaque in center.

3 Meanwhile, grate 2 teaspoons lemon peel from remaining lemon. Place in small bowl with butter, hot pepper sauce, if desired, and 1 tablespoon parsley; stir until well blended.

4 To serve, top each fillet with sauce mixture; sprinkle evenly with remaining 1 tablespoon parsley. Serve on lemon slices, if desired.

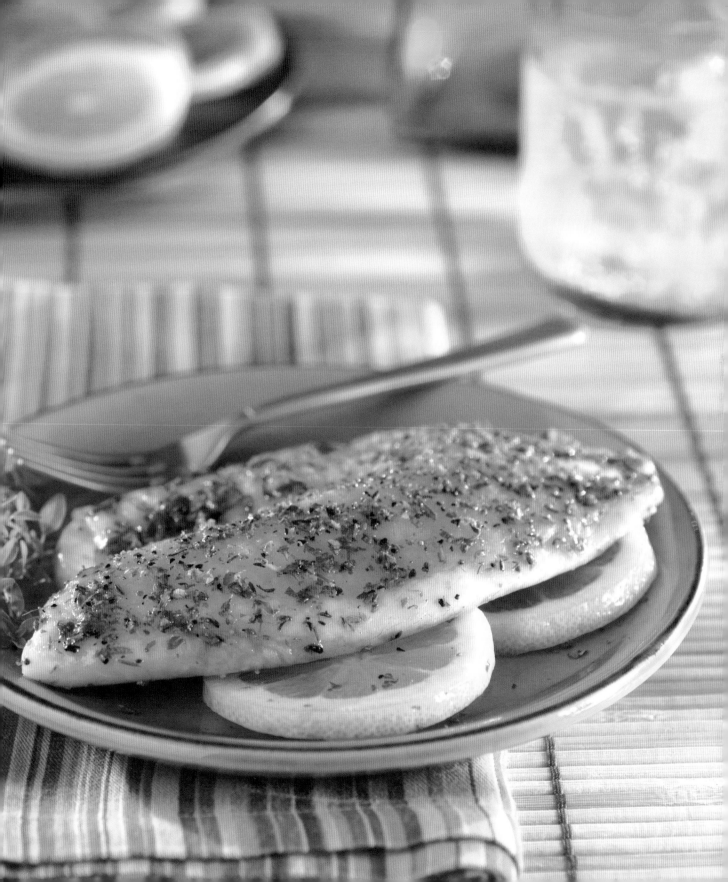

Szechuan Pork Stir-Fry over Spinach

MAKES 2 SERVINGS

2 teaspoons dark sesame oil, divided

¾ cup matchstick carrots

½ pound pork tenderloin, cut into thin strips

2 teaspoons minced fresh ginger

¼ teaspoon red pepper flakes

1 tablespoon reduced-sodium soy sauce

1 tablespoon mirin* or dry sherry

2 teaspoons cornstarch

8 ounces baby spinach

2 teaspoons sesame seeds, toasted**

Mirin, a sweet wine made from rice, is an essential flavoring in Japanese cuisine. It is available in Asian markets and the Asian or gourmet section of some supermarkets.

**To toast sesame seeds, spread in small skillet. Shake skillet over medium-low heat about 3 minutes or until seeds begin to pop and turn golden.*

1 Heat 1 teaspoon oil in large nonstick skillet over medium-high heat. Add carrots; stir-fry 3 minutes. Add pork, ginger and red pepper flakes; stir-fry 3 minutes or until pork is barely pink in center.

2 Whisk soy sauce, mirin and cornstarch in small bowl until well blended. Pour into skillet; stir-fry 1 minute or until thickened.

3 Heat remaining 1 teaspoon oil in medium saucepan over medium-high heat. Add spinach; cover and cook 1 minute or until spinach is barely wilted.

4 Arrange spinach on 2 serving plates. Top evenly with pork mixture; sprinkle evenly with sesame seeds.

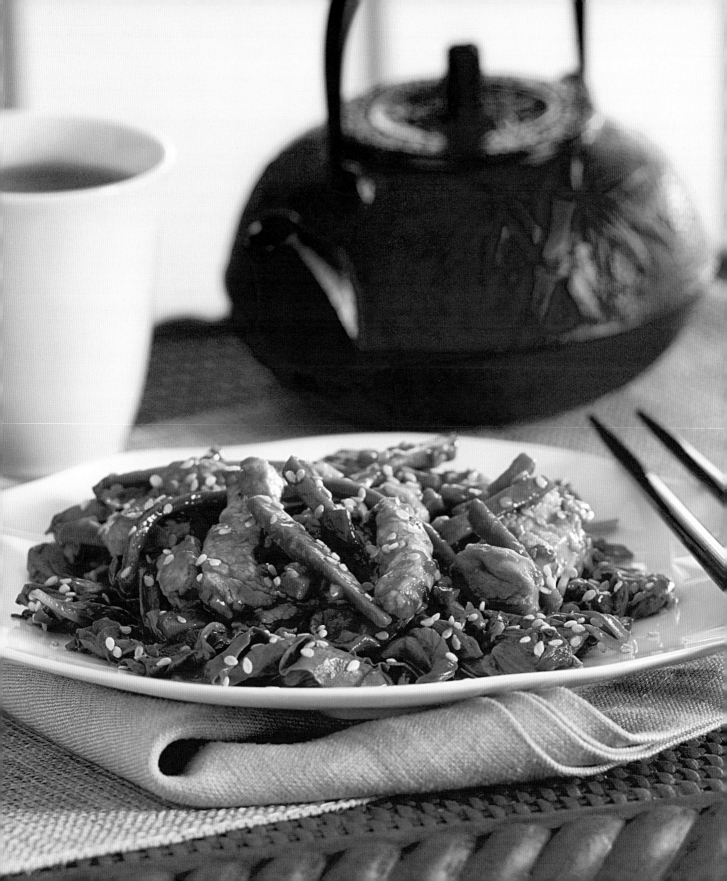

Vegetarian Stir-Fry

MAKES 4 SERVINGS

- 1 package (about 12 ounces) firm tofu
- ½ tablespoon salt-free seasoning blend
- ½ cup uncooked instant brown rice
- 1 bag (12 ounces) ready-to-use vegetable stir-fry mix
- ½ cup low-fat sesame ginger salad dressing

1 Preheat indoor-covered grill per grill instructions. Cut tofu into 4 (1-inch) slices. Sprinkle slices with seasoning blend. Grill 5 to 6 minutes. Set aside.

2 Prepare rice according to package instructions, omitting salt and fat. Cook vegetables in microwave according to package instructions. Toss vegetables with dressing in mixing bowl. Divide rice and vegetables among 4 plates. Top each with tofu slice.

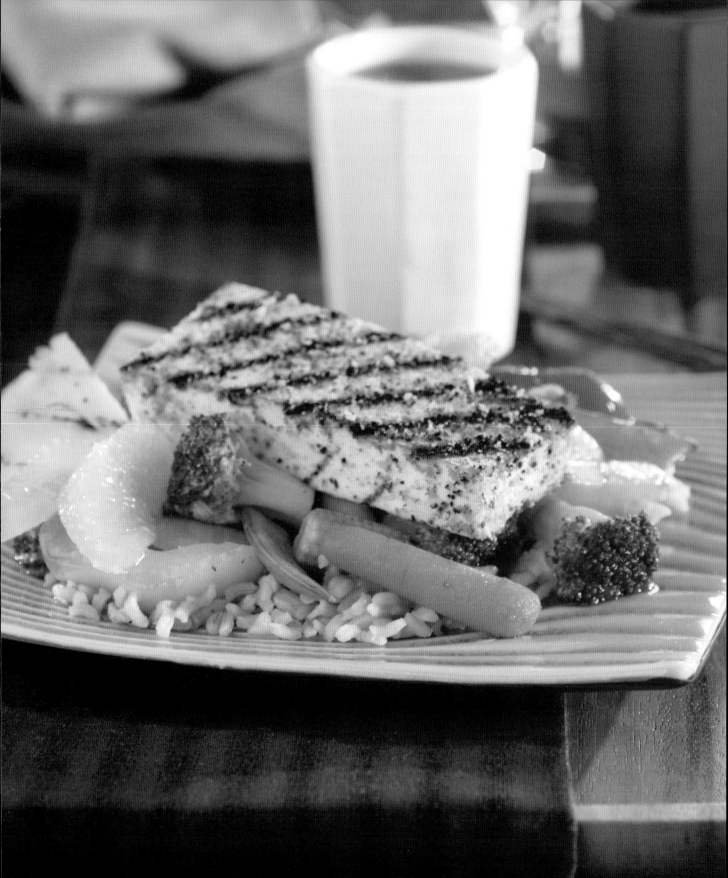

Scallops and Spinach over Potatoes

MAKES 4 SERVINGS

3 small or 2 medium Yukon Gold potatoes, cooked and diced

12 ounces bay scallops, rinsed and patted dry

¼ teaspoon salt

¼ teaspoon black pepper

4 cups baby spinach leaves

2 tablespoons minced fresh chives

1 teaspoon minced fresh tarragon

1 Spray large heavy skillet with nonstick cooking spray; heat over medium-high heat. Add potatoes; cook 10 to 12 minutes or until browned, stirring occasionally. Remove to serving dish; keep warm.

2 Spray same skillet with cooking spray; heat over medium-high heat. Add scallops, salt and pepper; cook and stir 3 minutes or until scallops begin to give off liquid. Add spinach, chives and tarragon. Reduce heat to medium; cook and stir 2 to 3 minutes or until scallops are cooked through and spinach is tender. Drain liquid from skillet. Spoon scallop mixture over potatoes; serve immediately.

TIP

Fresh herbs are very perishable so purchase them in small amounts. For short-term storage, place the herb stems in water. Cover leaves loosely with a plastic bag or plastic wrap and store in the refrigerator. They will last from 2 days (basil, chives, dill, mint, oregano) to 5 days (rosemary, sage, tarragon, thyme).

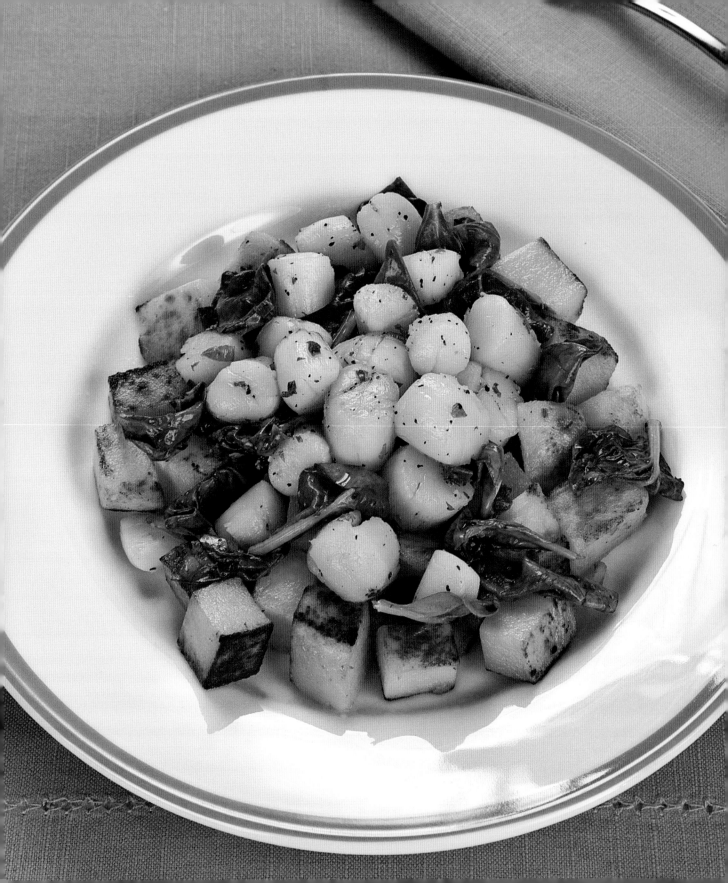

Szechuan Grilled Flank Steak

MAKES 4 TO 6 SERVINGS

- 1 beef flank steak
  (1¼ to 1½ pounds)
- ¼ cup seasoned rice
  wine vinegar
- ¼ cup soy sauce
- 2 tablespoons dark
  sesame oil
- 2 teaspoons minced
  fresh ginger
- ½ teaspoon garlic
  powder
- ½ teaspoon red pepper
  flakes
- ¼ cup water
- ½ cup thinly sliced
  green onions
  (green parts only)
- 2 to 3 teaspoons
  sesame seeds,
  toasted

  Hot cooked brown
  rice (optional)

1 Place steak in large resealable food storage bag. Combine vinegar, soy sauce, oil, ginger, garlic powder and red pepper flakes in small bowl; pour over steak. Seal bag; turn to coat. Marinate in refrigerator 3 hours, turning once.

2 Prepare grill for direct cooking. Remove steak from marinade; reserve marinade in small saucepan. Grill steak, uncovered, over medium heat 17 to 21 minutes for medium rare to medium or to desired doneness, turning once.

3 Add water to reserved marinade. Bring to a rolling boil over high heat. Boil for 1 minute. Slice steak against the grain into thin slices. Drizzle slices with boiled marinade. Sprinkle with green onions and sesame seeds. Serve with rice, if desired.

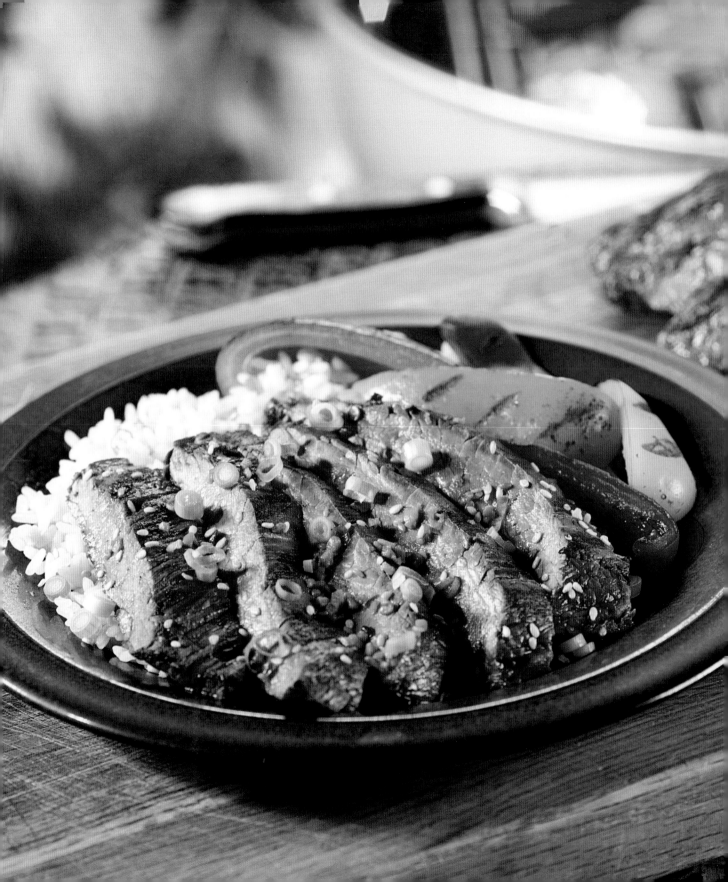

Tofu, Vegetable and Curry Stir-Fry

MAKES 4 SERVINGS

1 package (about 14 ounces) extra firm reduced-fat tofu, cut into ¾-inch cubes

¾ cup unsweetened canned coconut milk

2 tablespoons fresh lime juice

1 tablespoon curry powder

2 teaspoons dark sesame oil, divided

4 cups broccoli florets (1½ inch pieces)

2 medium red bell peppers, cut into short, thin strips

¼ teaspoon salt

Hot cooked brown rice (optional)

1 Press tofu cubes between layers of paper towels to remove excess moisture. Combine coconut milk, lime juice and curry powder in medium bowl.

2 Heat 1 teaspoon oil in large nonstick skillet over medium heat. Add tofu; cook 10 minutes or until lightly browned on all sides, turning cubes often. Remove to plate; set aside.

3 Add remaining 1 teaspoon oil to skillet; increase heat to high. Add broccoli and bell peppers; stir-fry about 5 minutes or until vegetables are crisp-tender. Stir in tofu and coconut milk mixture; cook and stir until mixture comes to a boil. Stir in salt. Serve immediately with rice, if desired.

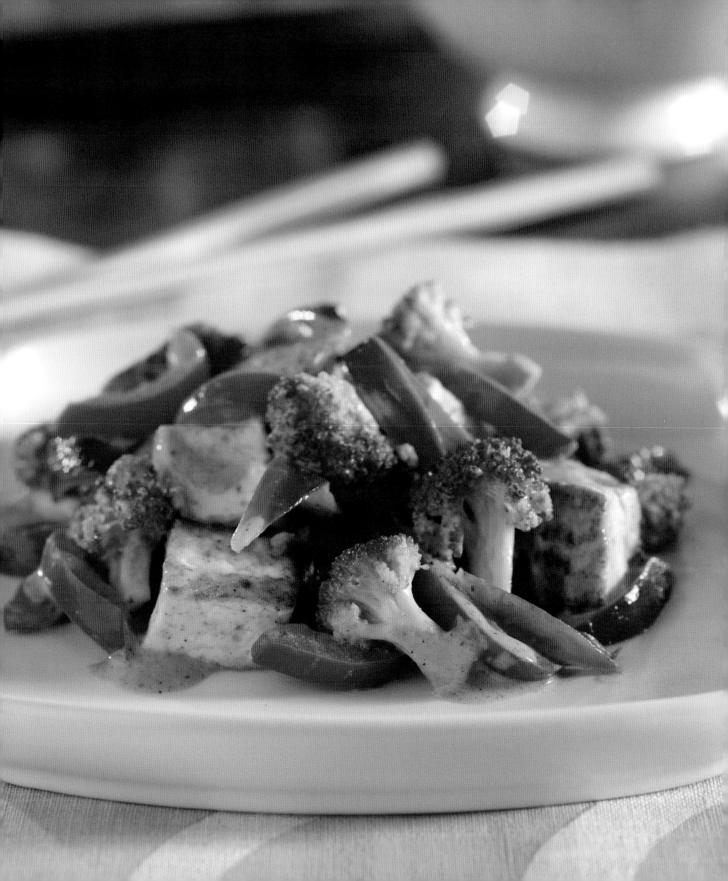

Miso Salmon & Spinach

MAKES 4 SERVINGS

½ **cup sake**

¼ **cup white miso***

¼ **cup mirin**

4 **boneless skinless salmon fillets or steaks (about 5 ounces each)**

1 **bag (10 ounces) baby spinach**

Soy sauce

2 **teaspoons sesame seeds, toasted**

A fermented soybean paste used frequently in Japanese cooking. Miso comes in many varieties; the light yellow miso, usually labeled "white" is the mildest. Look for it in tubs or plastic pouches in the produce section or Asian aisle of the supermarket.

1 Combine sake, miso and mirin in large deep skillet or Dutch oven. Bring to a boil over high heat. Reduce heat to medium; add salmon. Simmer, uncovered, 4 minutes. Turn salmon over; simmer 3 to 4 minutes more or until salmon is opaque in center. Transfer salmon to plate and keep warm.

2 Add spinach in two batches to liquid in skillet; cook 2 minutes or until spinach is wilted. Remove spinach with slotted spoon and keep warm.

3 Turn heat to high and bring liquid to a gentle boil. Cook 1 to 2 minutes or until sauce is reduced to about ¼ cup. Season with soy sauce.

4 Serve salmon over spinach; drizzle with sauce and sprinkle with sesame seeds.

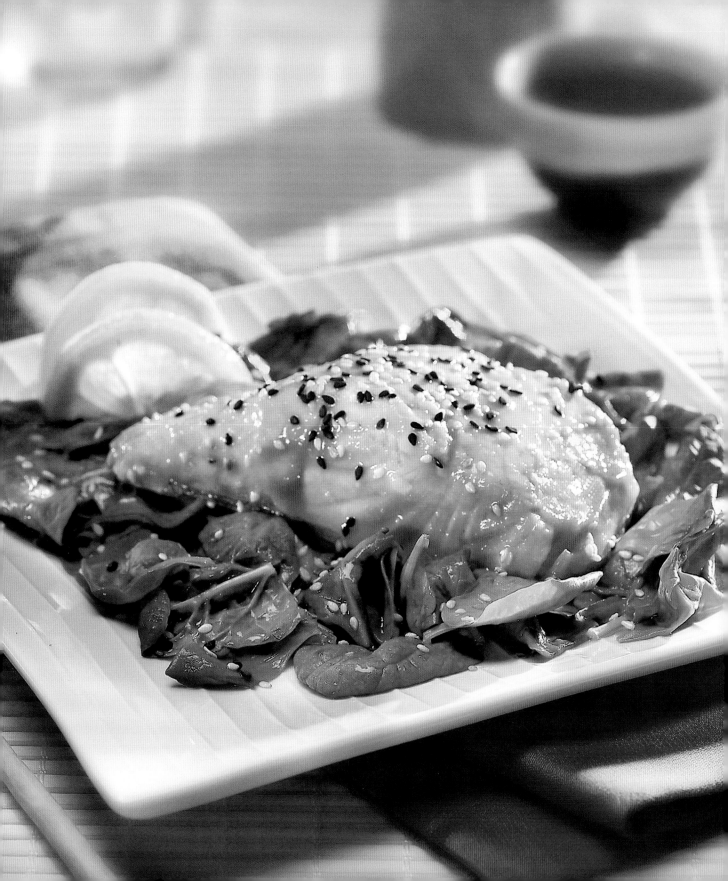

Noodles with Baby Shrimp

MAKES 4 TO 6 SERVINGS

1 package (3¾ ounces) cellophane noodles

3 green onions (green parts only)

1 tablespoon olive oil

1 package (16 ounces) frozen mixed vegetables (such as cauliflower, broccoli and carrots)

1 cup vegetable broth

8 ounces cooked frozen baby shrimp

1 tablespoon soy sauce

2 teaspoons dark sesame oil

¼ teaspoon black pepper

1 Place noodles in large bowl. Cover with boiling water; let stand 10 to 15 minutes or just until softened. Drain noodles. Cut noodles into 5- or 6-inch pieces; set aside. Cut green onions into 1-inch pieces.

2 Heat wok or large skillet over high heat about 1 minute or until hot. Drizzle olive oil into wok; heat 30 seconds. Add green onions; stir-fry 1 minute. Add mixed vegetables; stir-fry 2 minutes. Add broth; bring to a boil. Reduce heat to low; cover and cook 5 minutes or until vegetables are crisp-tender.

3 Add shrimp to wok; cook just until thawed. Stir in noodles, soy sauce, sesame oil and pepper; stir-fry until heated through.

TIP

Cellophane noodles are also called bean thread noodles or glass noodles. These clear, thin noodles are made from mung bean starch and so are gluten-free. They are sold in packages of 6 to 8 tangled bunches in the Asian section of the supermarket.

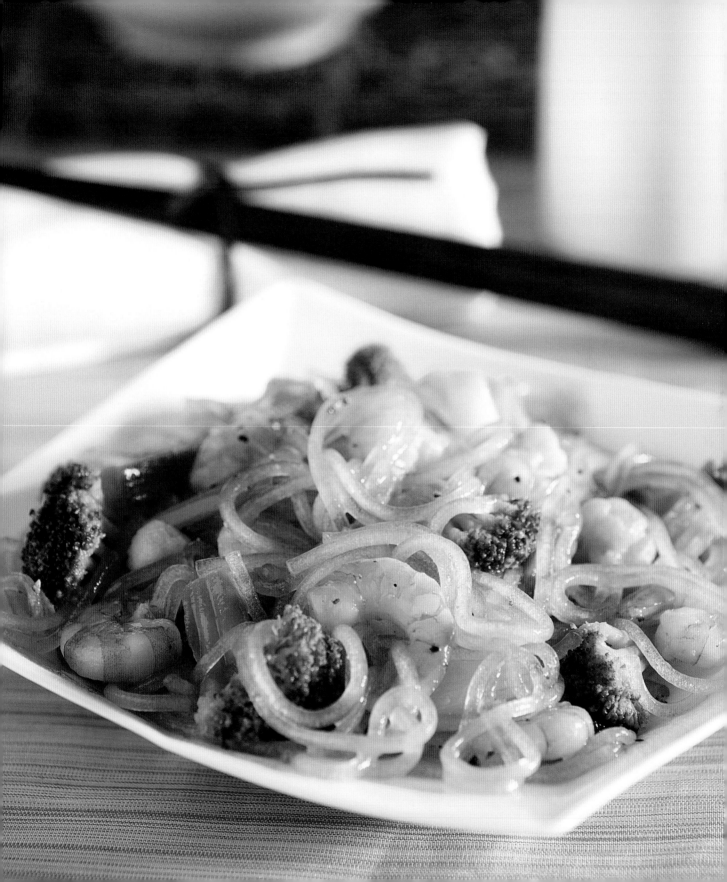

Pan-Seared Tuna with Spicy Horseradish Sauce

MAKES 4 SERVINGS

SPICY HORSERADISH SAUCE

- ½ **cup fat-free plain Greek yogurt**
- 1 **tablespoon water**
- 2 **teaspoons prepared horseradish**
- 1 **teaspoon Dijon mustard**
- ½ **teaspoon garlic powder**
- ½ **teaspoon dried rosemary**
- ½ **teaspoon salt**

- 4 **fresh tuna steaks (4 ounces each), rinsed and patted dry**
- 2 **teaspoons no-salt-added steak seasoning blend**
- 2 **tablespoons finely chopped parsley**

1 Combine yogurt, water, horseradish, mustard, garlic powder, rosemary and salt in small bowl; set aside.

2 Sprinkle both sides of tuna with steak seasoning blend, pressing down with fingertips to adhere.

3 Coat grill pan with nonstick cooking spray; heat over medium-high heat. Cook tuna 1½ minutes on each side. *(Do not overcook or tuna will be tough and dry.)* Remove from pan; serve topped with parsley and Spicy Horseradish Sauce.

TIP

Serve this recipe with green vegetables for an overall nutritious meal.

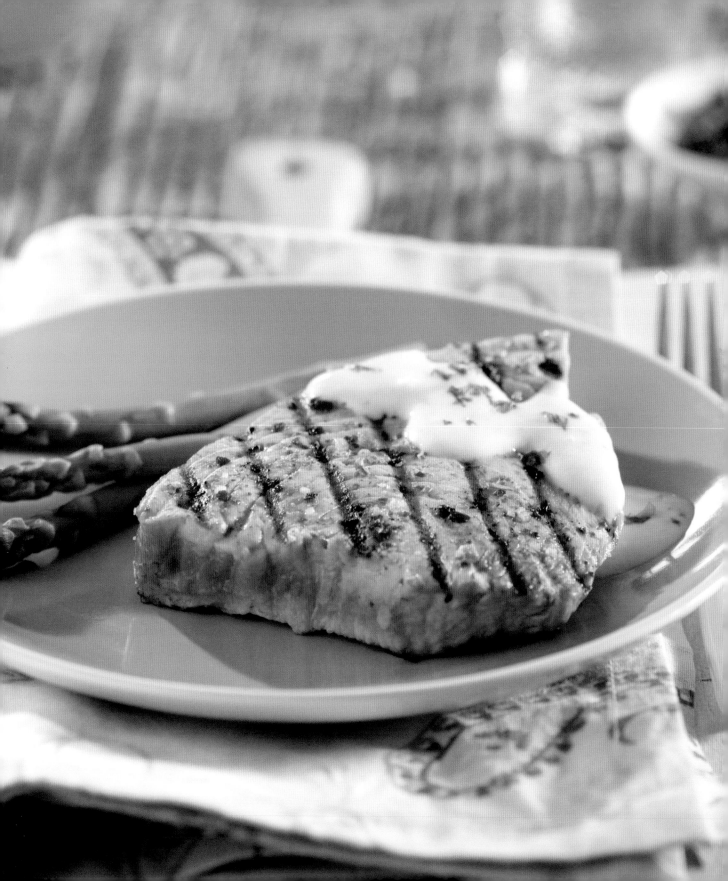

Shrimp and Veggie Skillet Toss

MAKES 4 SERVINGS

¼ cup soy sauce

2 tablespoons lime juice

1 tablespoon sesame oil

1 teaspoon grated fresh ginger

⅛ teaspoon red pepper flakes

32 medium raw shrimp (about 8 ounces total), peeled, deveined, rinsed and patted dry (with tails on)

2 medium zucchini, cut in half lengthwise and thinly sliced

6 green onions (green parts only)

12 grape tomatoes

1 Whisk soy sauce, lime juice, oil, ginger and red pepper flakes in small bowl; set aside.

2 Spray large nonstick skillet with nonstick cooking spray; heat over medium-high heat. Add shrimp; cook and stir 3 minutes or until shrimp are pink and opaque. Remove from skillet.

3 Spray same skillet with cooking spray. Add zucchini; cook and stir 4 to 6 minutes or just until crisp-tender. Add green onions and tomatoes; cook 1 to 2 minutes. Add shrimp, cook 1 minute. Transfer to large bowl.

4 Add soy sauce mixture to skillet; bring to a boil. Remove from heat. Stir in shrimp and vegetables; gently toss.

NOTE

Shrimp are very low in calories and fat, and high in protein. They're also a good source of vitamin D and vitamin B12. All seafood are very sensitive to temperature, so return shrimp to refrigerator as soon as possible after purchasing.

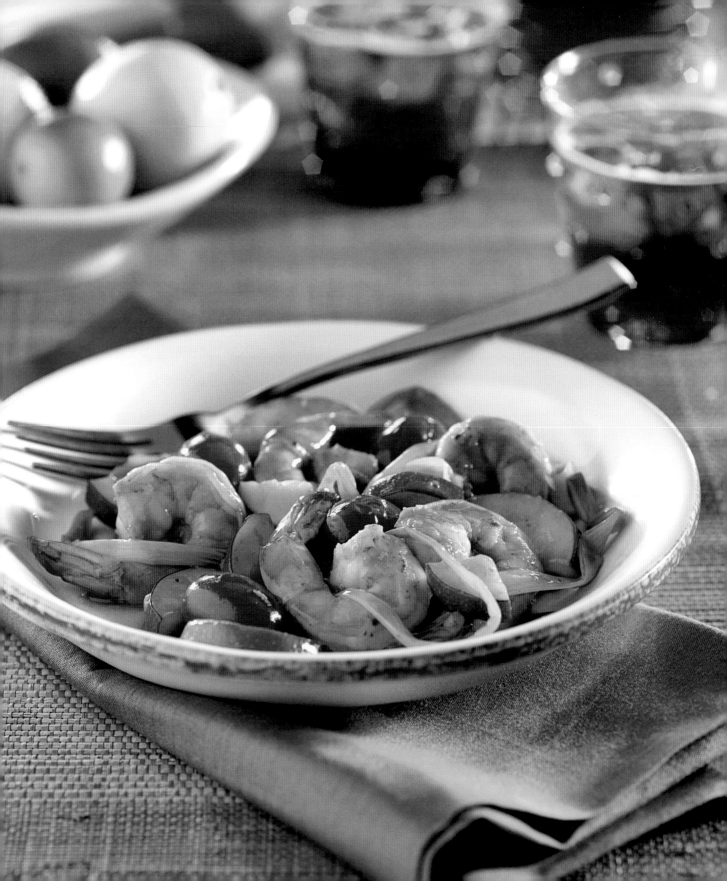

Curried Shrimp & Vegetable Noodle Bowl

MAKES 2 SERVINGS

 2 **ounces thin rice noodles (rice vermicelli)**

 1 **teaspoon canola oil**

 ¾ **cup broccoli**

 ¼ **cup snow peas, diagonally halved**

 4 **ounces medium raw shrimp, peeled and deveined**

 1 **cup packed chopped bok choy leaves**

 ⅓ **cup unsweetened canned coconut milk**

 1½ **tablespoons red curry paste***

 2 **tablespoons chopped fresh cilantro**

*Red curry paste can be found in jars in the Asian food section of the supermarket. Spice levels can vary between brands. Start with 1 tablespoon, then add more as desired.

1 Place rice noodles in medium bowl. Cover with hot water; let stand 15 minutes or until tender. Drain. When cool enough to handle, cut noodles into 3-inch lengths.

2 Meanwhile, heat oil in large nonstick skillet over medium heat. Add broccoli and snow peas; stir-fry 3 minutes. Add shrimp and bok choy; stir-fry 5 minutes or until shrimp are pink and opaque and vegetables are crisp-tender. Add coconut milk and curry paste; stir-fry 1 to 2 minutes or until sauce is thickened.

3 Add noodles to mixture; toss well.

4 Divide mixture evenly among 2 bowls. Top evenly with cilantro.

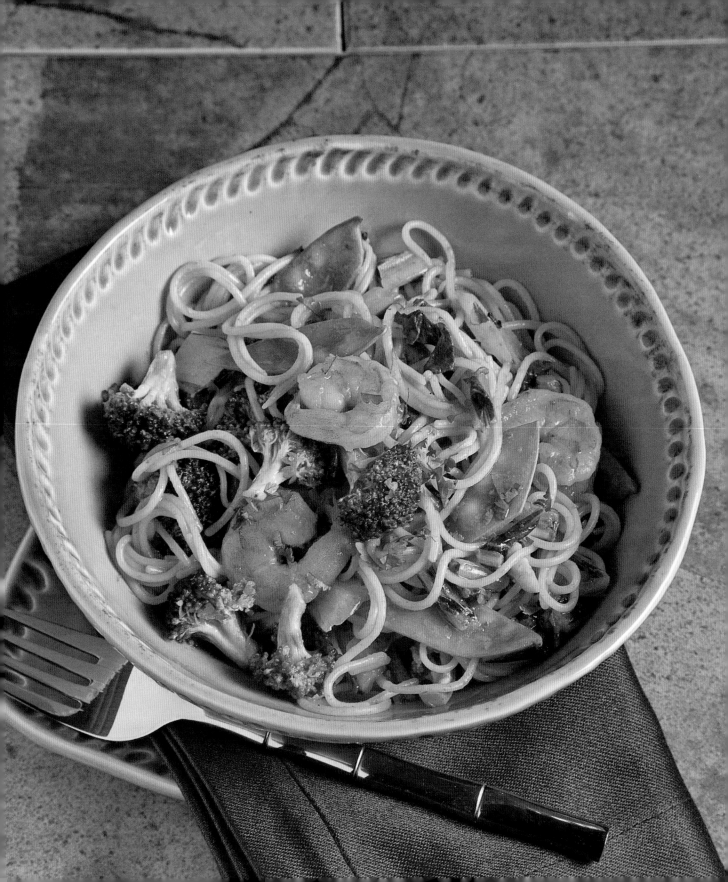

Sesame-Garlic Flank Steak

MAKES 4 SERVINGS

1 **beef flank steak (about 1¼ pounds)**

2 **tablespoons soy sauce**

2 **tablespoons hoisin sauce**

1 **tablespoon dark sesame oil**

½ **teaspoon garlic powder**

1 Score steak lightly with sharp knife in diamond pattern on both sides; place in large resealable food storage bag. Combine soy sauce, hoisin sauce, sesame oil and garlic powder in small bowl; pour over steak. Seal bag; turn to coat. Marinate in refrigerator at least 2 hours or up to 24 hours, turning once.

2 Prepare grill for direct cooking. Remove steak from marinade; reserve marinade. Grill steak, covered, over medium heat 13 to 18 minutes for medium rare (145°F) to medium (160°F) or to desired doneness, turning and brushing with marinade halfway through cooking time. Discard remaining marinade.

3 Transfer steak to cutting board; carve across the grain into thin slices.

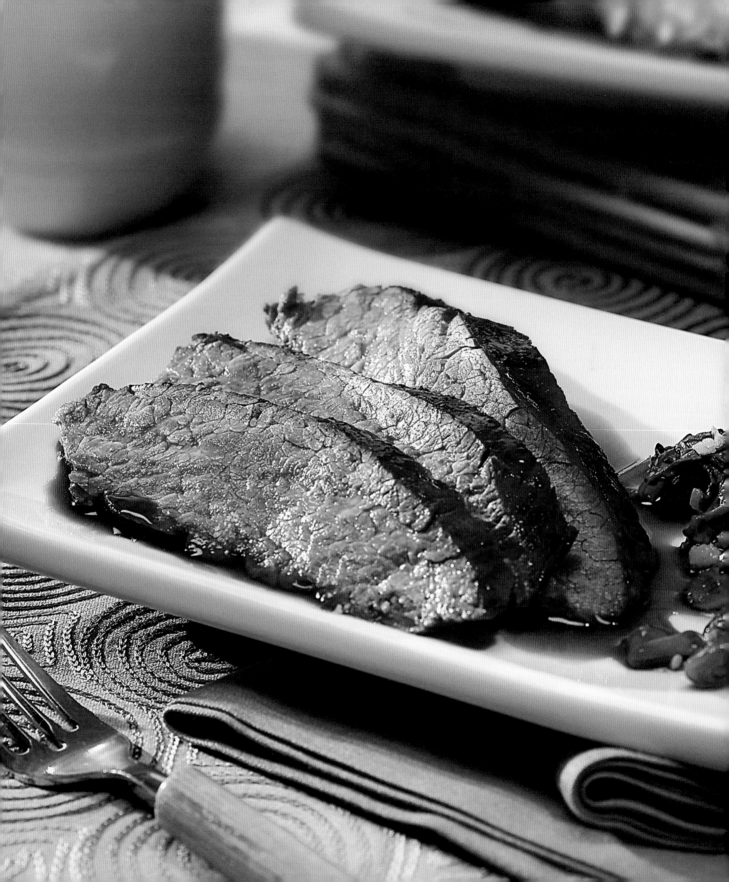

Shrimp, Chicken and Cucumber Salad

MAKES 4 SERVINGS

1 quart plus
  3 tablespoons
  water, divided

3 chicken thighs
  (about 14 ounces)

2 medium cucumbers,
  cut in half
  lengthwise, seeded
  and thinly sliced

1 large carrot, cut into
  matchstick-size
  strips

1 teaspoon salt

2 tablespoons fish
  sauce

1 tablespoon sugar

1½ tablespoons fresh
  lime juice

½ teaspoon garlic
  powder

4 jumbo cooked
  shrimp, peeled
  and deveined
  (with tails on)

1 tablespoon chopped
  fresh cilantro

1 tablespoon chopped
  fresh mint

1 tablespoon chopped
  fresh basil

1 tablespoon chopped
  green onion
  (green parts only)

1 Heat 1 quart water in medium saucepan over high heat to boiling. Add chicken. Reduce heat to low; simmer, covered, until tender, about 25 minutes. Drain chicken; let stand until cool enough to handle. Skin and debone chicken; cut into ¼-inch cubes.

2 Meanwhile, combine cucumbers and carrot in large bowl; sprinkle with salt. Toss to mix well; let stand 15 minutes.

3 For dressing, combine remaining 3 tablespoons water, fish sauce, sugar, lime juice and garlic powder in small bowl; stir until sugar is dissolved.

4 Squeeze cucumber mixture to extract liquid; discard liquid.

5 Combine cucumber mixture and chicken in medium bowl; drizzle with dressing. Toss to mix well; refrigerate, covered, 30 minutes to 2 hours.

6 Cut shrimp in half lengthwise, leaving tails attached. Mix cilantro, mint, basil and green onion in small bowl.

7 Transfer salad mixture to serving dish. Garnish with shrimp; top with mixed herbs.

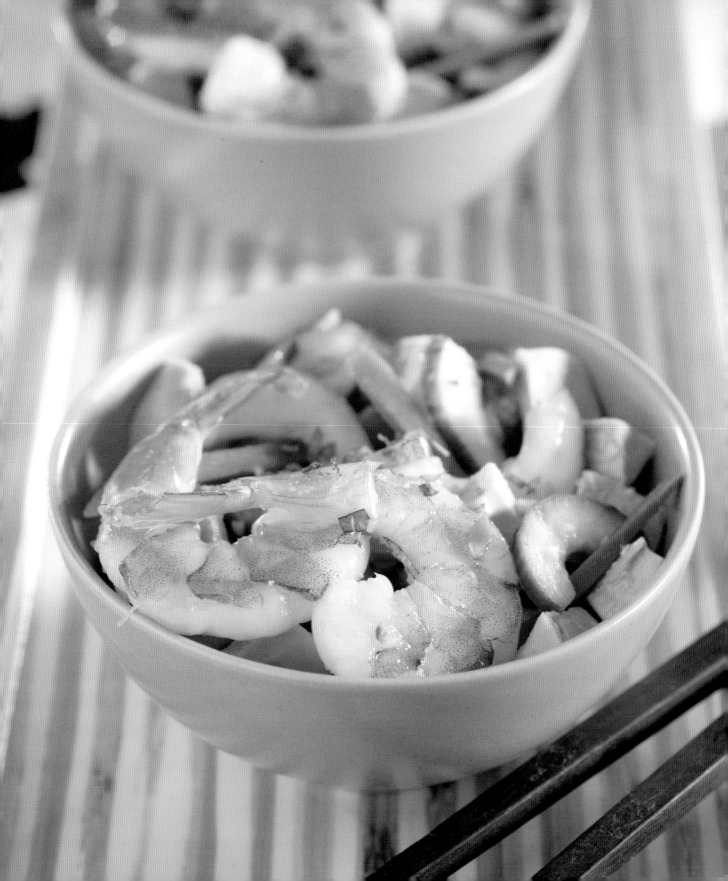

Herbed Lamb Chops

MAKES 4 TO 6 SERVINGS

- ⅓ **cup vegetable oil**
- ⅓ **cup red wine vinegar**
- 2 **tablespoons soy sauce**
- 1 **tablespoon lemon juice**
- ½ **teaspoon garlic powder**
- 1 **teaspoon salt**
- 1 **teaspoon chopped fresh oregano *or* ¼ teaspoon dried oregano**
- 1 **teaspoon dried rosemary**
- 1 **teaspoon ground mustard**
- ½ **teaspoon white pepper**
- 8 **lamb loin chops, 1 inch thick (about 2 pounds)**

1 Combine all ingredients except lamb in large resealable food storage bag. Reserve ½ cup marinade in small bowl. Add lamb to remaining marinade. Seal bag; turn to coat. Marinate in refrigerator at least 1 hour.

2 Prepare grill for direct cooking over medium-high heat.

3 Remove lamb from marinade; discard marinade. Grill lamb over medium-high heat 8 minutes or to desired doneness, turning once and basting often with reserved ½ cup marinade. Do not baste during last 5 minutes of cooking. Discard any remaining marinade.

HINT

Substitute ¼ to ½ teaspoon dried herbs for each teaspoon of fresh herbs.

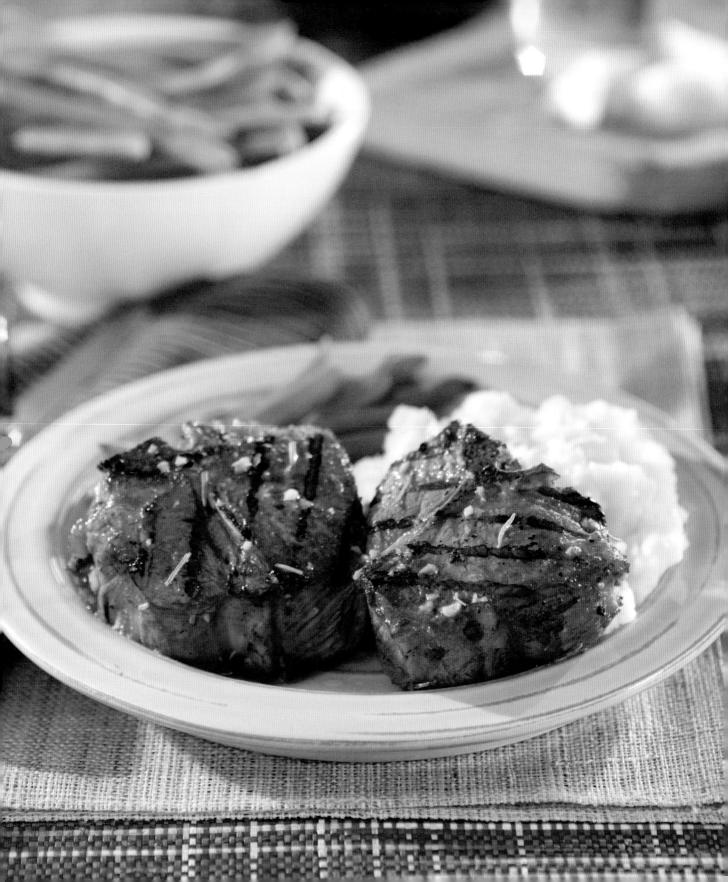

Hip Hop Hash

MAKES 4 SERVINGS

1 tablespoon olive oil

1 tablespoon sweet rice flour (mochiko)

⅓ cup beef broth

1 teaspoon Worcestershire sauce

1 pound beef pot roast, cooked and diced

1 medium sweet potato (about 12 ounces), peeled and diced

1 stalk celery, diced

½ cup corn

¼ cup diced red or green bell pepper

1 Heat oil in large skillet over medium heat. Whisk in rice flour; cook 2 minutes, stirring constantly. Whisk in broth and Worcestershire sauce; bring to a simmer.

2 Add beef, sweet potato, celery, corn and bell pepper. Return to a simmer; cover and cook 12 minutes or until vegetables are tender.

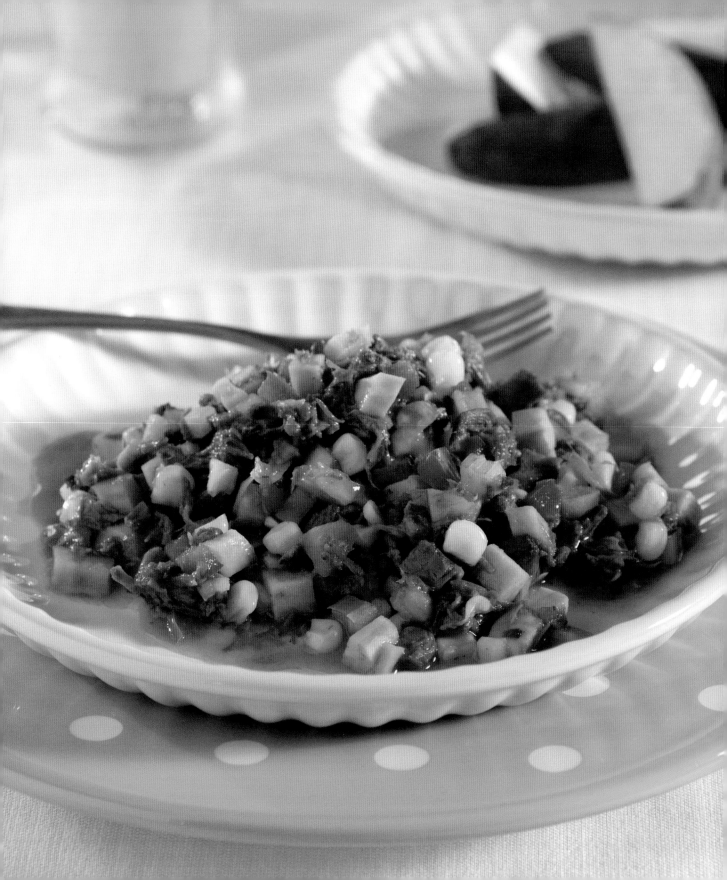

Lemony Seasoned Tilapia Fillets

MAKES 4 SERVINGS

2 teaspoons dried oregano

1 teaspoon grated lemon peel

1 tablespoon lemon juice

Salt and black pepper, to taste

4 tilapia fillets (about 1 pound)

2 tablespoons olive oil

1 Combine oregano, lemon peel, lemon juice, salt and pepper in small bowl. Brush both sides of tilapia with mixture.

2 Heat oil in large skillet over medium-high heat. Cook tilapia 4 to 5 minutes; turn. Cook 4 to 5 minutes or until fish begins to flake when tested with fork.

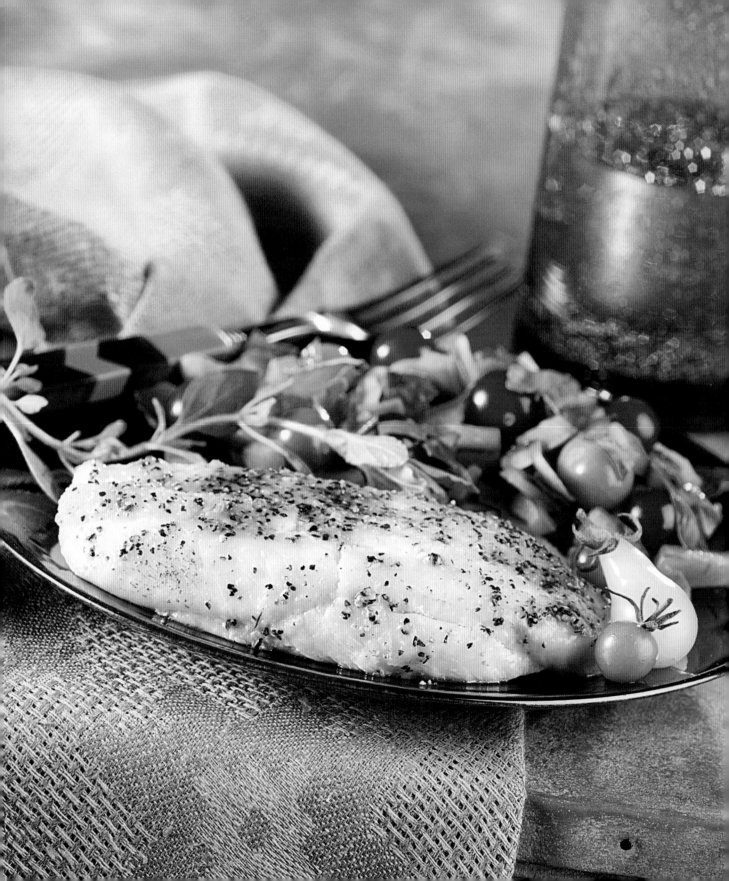

Mediterranean Tuna Salad

MAKES 4 SERVINGS

- ½ **cup diced tomato**
- 1 **tablespoon olive oil**
- 1 **tablespoon lemon juice**
- 2 **teaspoons Dijon mustard**
- ½ **teaspoon garlic powder**
- ¼ **teaspoon salt**
- ¼ **teaspoon dried basil**
- 2 **cans (6 ounces each) solid white tuna packed in water, drained and flaked**
- ½ **cup diced celery**
- ⅓ **cup chopped fresh basil**
- **Red leaf lettuce leaves**
- ½ **pound steamed green beans**
- 1 **medium red bell pepper, seeded and cut into strips**
- 8 **cherry tomatoes, halved**

1 Combine diced tomato, oil, lemon juice, mustard, garlic powder, salt and dried basil in large bowl; let stand 5 minutes. Stir in tuna, celery and fresh basil. Refrigerate, covered, 1 to 2 hours to allow flavors to blend, stirring once.

2 Line serving platter with lettuce leaves. Mound tuna salad in center; surround with green beans, bell pepper and cherry tomatoes.

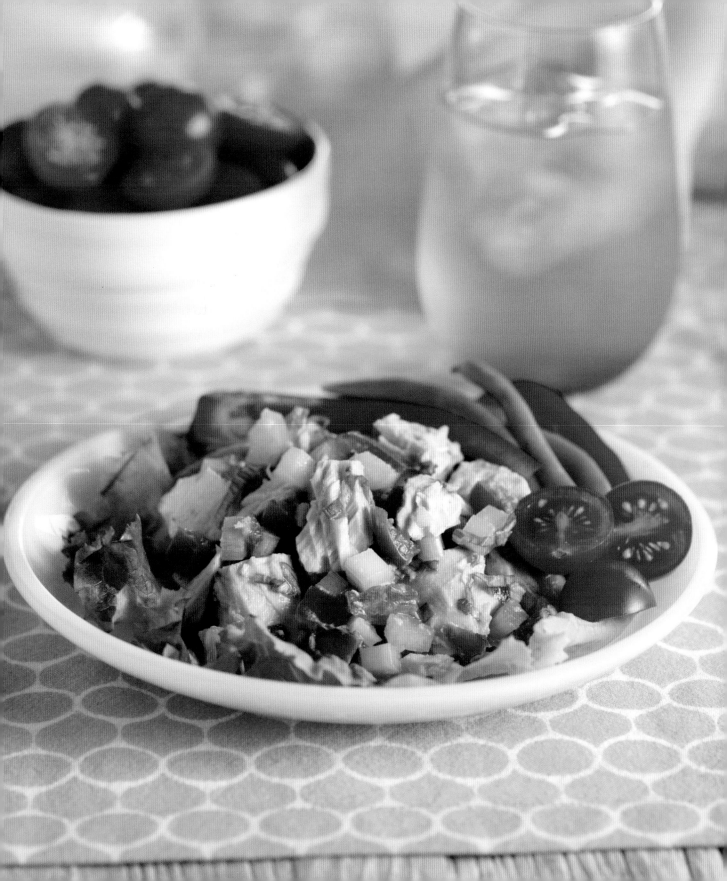

Cilantro-Stuffed Chicken Breasts

MAKES 4 SERVINGS

½ **teaspoon garlic powder**

1 **cup packed fresh cilantro leaves**

1 **tablespoon plus 2 teaspoons soy sauce, divided**

1 **tablespoon olive oil**

4 **chicken breast halves with skin on (about 1¼ pounds)**

1 **tablespoon dark sesame oil**

1 Preheat oven to 350°F. Combine garlic powder and cilantro in food processor. Add 2 teaspoons soy sauce and olive oil; process until paste forms.

2 With rubber spatula or fingers, distribute about 1 tablespoon cilantro mixture evenly under skin of each chicken breast half, taking care not to puncture skin.

3 Place chicken on rack in shallow, foil-lined baking pan. Combine remaining 1 tablespoon soy sauce and sesame oil in small bowl. Brush half of mixture evenly over chicken. Bake 25 minutes; brush remaining soy sauce mixture evenly over chicken. Bake 10 minutes or until juices run clear.

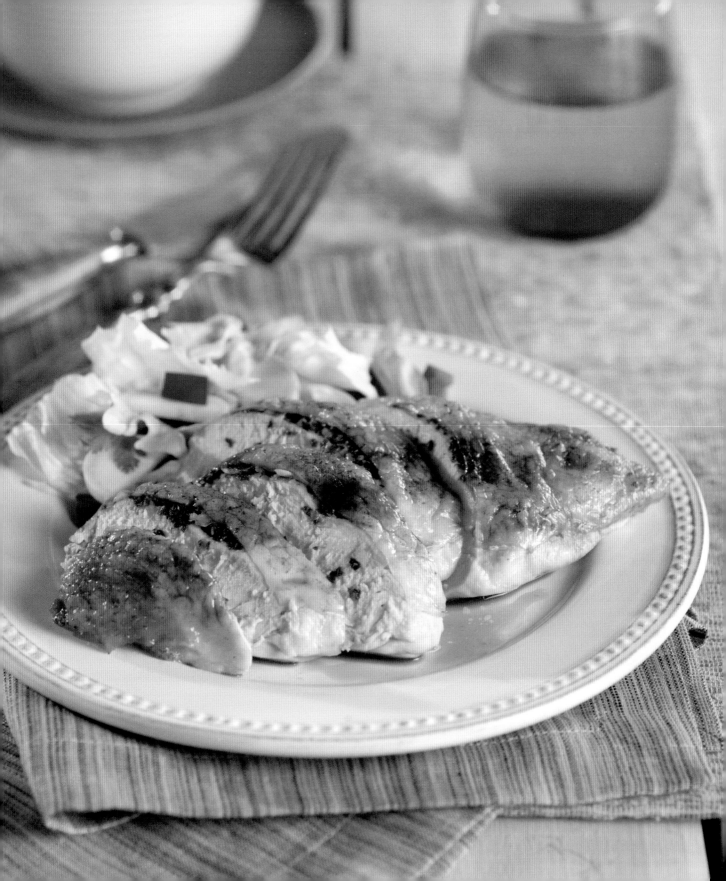

Crab Spinach Salad with Tarragon Dressing

MAKES 4 SERVINGS

12 ounces coarsely flaked cooked crabmeat *or* 2 packages (6 ounces each) frozen crabmeat, thawed and drained

½ cup chopped tomatoes

1 cup sliced cucumber

2 tablespoons sliced red onion

¼ cup fat-free salad dressing

¼ cup plain nonfat Greek yogurt

¼ cup chopped fresh parsley

2 tablespoons fat-free (skim) milk

2 teaspoons chopped fresh tarragon *or* ½ teaspoon dried tarragon

½ teaspoon garlic powder

¼ teaspoon hot pepper sauce

8 cups fresh spinach

1 Combine crabmeat, tomatoes, cucumber and onion in medium bowl. Combine salad dressing, yogurt, parsley, milk, tarragon, garlic powder and hot pepper sauce in small bowl.

2 Line 4 salad plates with spinach. Place crabmeat mixture on spinach; drizzle with dressing.

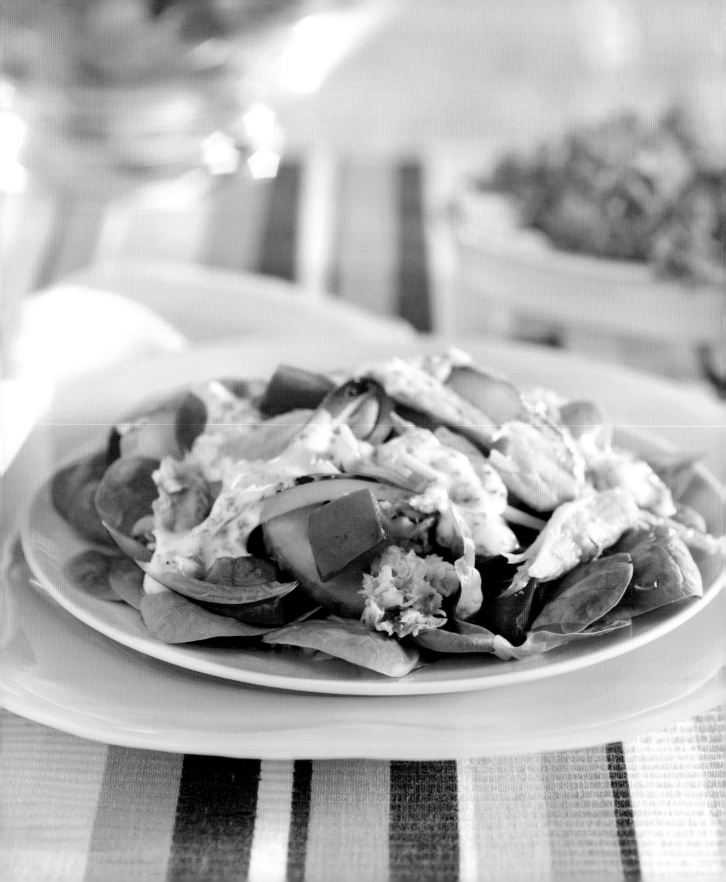

Thai Grilled Beef Salad

MAKES 4 SERVINGS

3 tablespoons Thai seasoning, divided

1 beef flank steak (about 1 pound)

2 tablespoons chopped fresh cilantro

2 tablespoons chopped fresh basil

1 red jalapeño pepper,* seeded and sliced into thin slivers *or* 2 red Thai peppers

1 tablespoon finely chopped lemongrass

Juice of 1 lime

1 tablespoon fish sauce

1 large carrot, grated

1 cucumber, chopped

4 cups assorted salad greens

Jalapeño peppers and Thai chili peppers and can sting and irritate the skin, so wear rubber gloves when handling peppers and do not touch your eyes.

1 Prepare grill for direct grilling.

2 Sprinkle 1 tablespoon Thai seasoning over beef; turn to coat. Cover and marinate 15 minutes. Place steak on grid over medium heat. Grill, uncovered, 17 to 21 minutes for medium rare (135°F.) to medium (145°F.) or until desired doneness, turning once. Cool 10 minutes.

3 Meanwhile, combine remaining 2 tablespoons Thai seasoning, cilantro, basil, jalapeño pepper, lemongrass, lime juice and fish sauce in medium bowl; mix well.

4 Thinly slice beef across grain. Add beef, carrot and cucumber to dressing; toss to coat. Arrange on bed of greens.

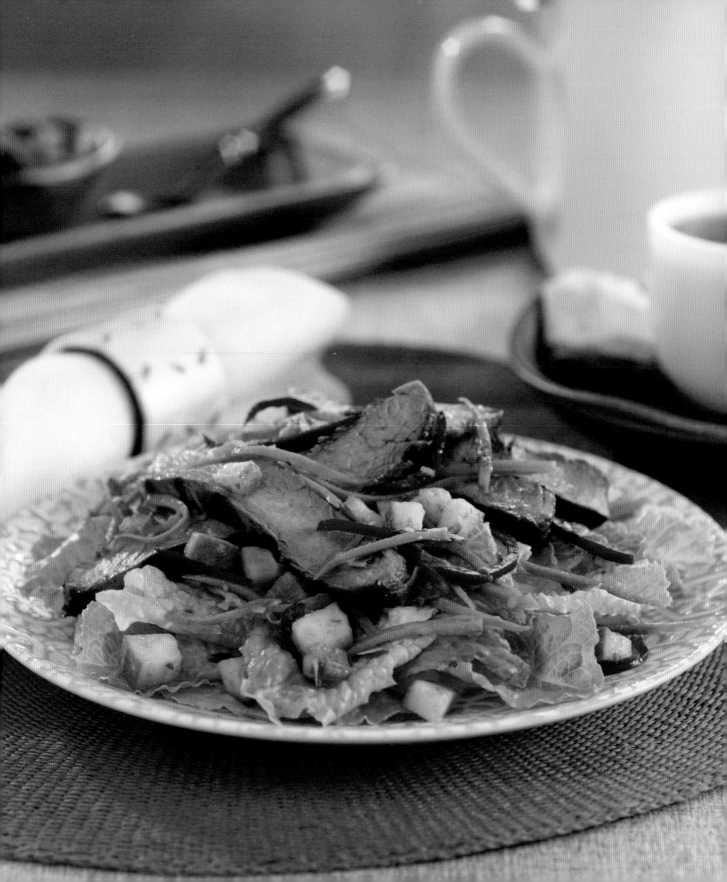

Chicken Kabobs over Quinoa

MAKES 4 SERVINGS

½ **cup uncooked quinoa**

1 **cup water**

1 **jalapeño pepper,***
  seeded and finely
  chopped (optional)

3 **teaspoons grated**
  lemon peel,
  divided

½ **teaspoon salt, divided**

1 **pound skinless**
  boneless chicken
  breasts, cut into
  cubes

2 **teaspoons chicken**
  seasoning blend

4 **asparagus spears,**
  trimmed and
  sliced

8 **grape tomatoes**

2 **green onions (green**
  parts only), sliced

2 **tablespoons lemon**
  juice

2 **tablespoons extra**
  virgin olive oil

¼ **cup chopped fresh**
  cilantro

**Jalapeño peppers can
sting and irritate the skin,
so wear rubber gloves
when handling peppers
and do not touch your
eyes.*

1 Place quinoa in fine-mesh strainer; rinse well under cold running water. Bring 1 cup water to a boil in small saucepan; stir in quinoa. Reduce heat to low; cover and simmer 10 to 15 minutes or until quinoa is tender and water is absorbed. Remove from heat. Stir in jalapeño pepper, if desired, 2 teaspoons lemon peel and ¼ teaspoon salt. Keep warm.

2 Meanwhile, soak 8 (12-inch) wooden skewers in cold water 10 to 20 minutes. Sprinkle chicken cubes with seasoning blend. Thread asparagus, chicken, tomatoes and green onions onto skewers.

3 Combine lemon juice, remaining 1 teaspoon lemon peel, oil and remaining ¼ teaspoon salt in small bowl. Reserve half of mixture; brush remaining mixture over chicken and vegetable kabobs.

4 Oil grid. Prepare grill for direct cooking. Grill skewers 3 to 4 minutes on each side or until chicken is cooked through.

5 Brush skewers with reserved lemon juice mixture. Stir cilantro into quinoa; serve with skewers.

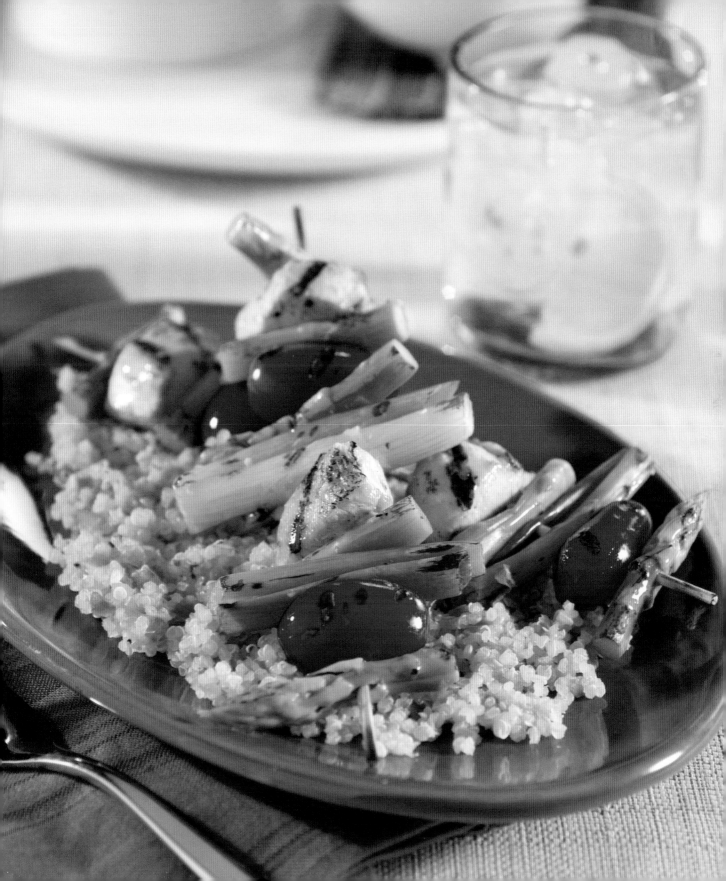

Spinach and Feta Farro Stuffed Peppers

MAKES 6 SERVINGS

1 tablespoon olive oil

1 package (5 ounces) baby spinach

½ cup sliced green onions (green parts only)

1 tablespoon chopped fresh oregano

1 package (8.8 ounces) quick-cooking farro, prepared according to package directions using vegetable broth in place of water

½ cup diced tomatoes

⅛ teaspoon black pepper

1 container (4 ounces) crumbled feta cheese, divided

3 large bell peppers, halved lengthwise, cores and ribs removed

1 Preheat oven to 350°F.

2 Heat oil in large skillet over medium-high heat. Add spinach, green onions and oregano; cook and stir 3 minutes. Stir in farro, tomatoes, black pepper and ½ cup cheese.

3 Spoon farro mixture into bell pepper halves (about ¾ cup each); place in shallow baking pan. Pour ¼ cup water into bottom of pan; cover with foil.

4 Bake 30 minutes or until bell peppers are crisp-tender and filling is heated through. Sprinkle with remaining cheese.

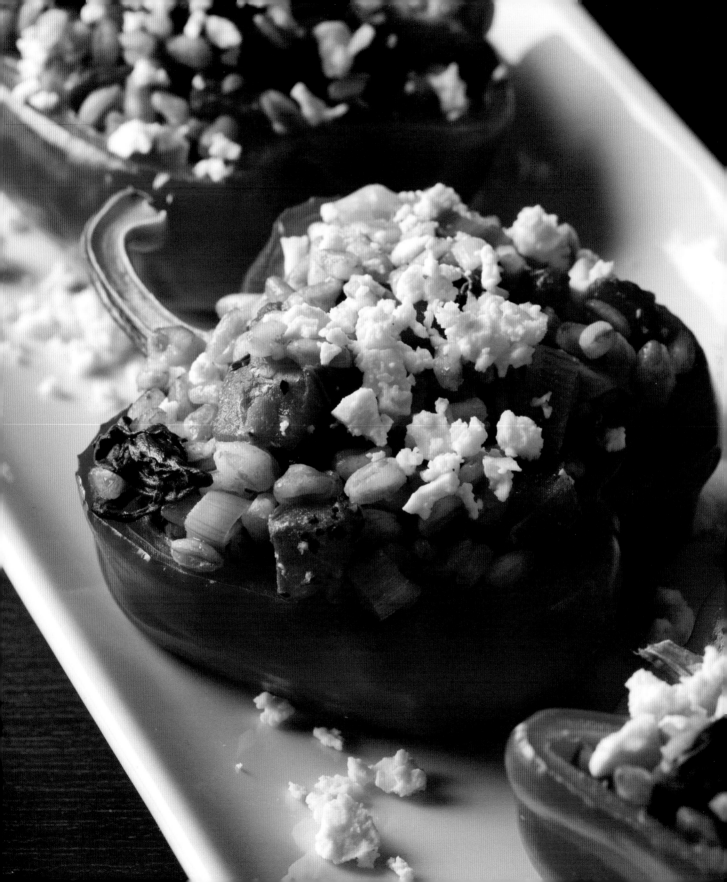

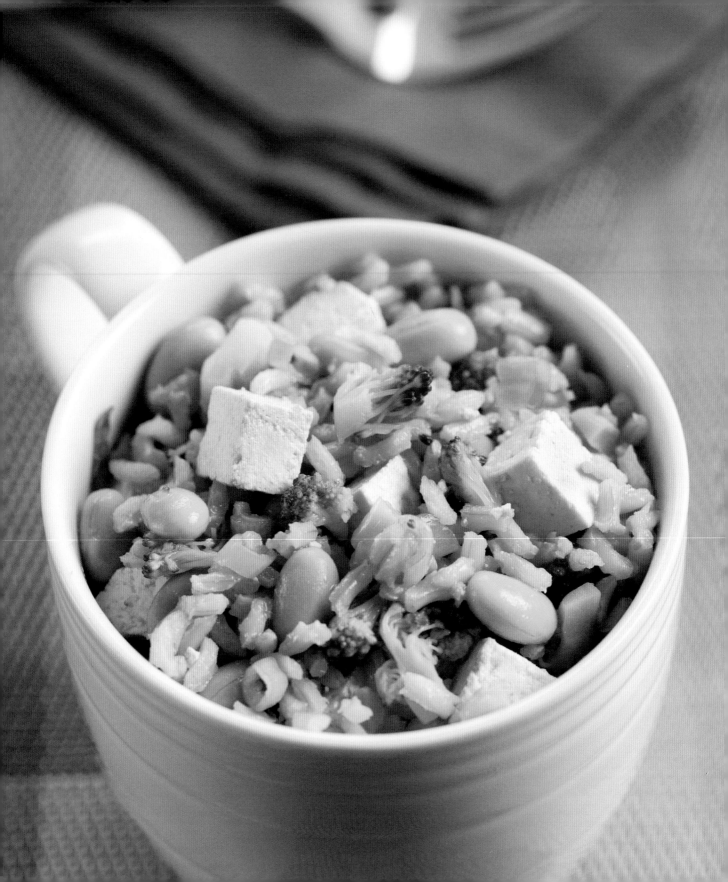

SOUPS & SIDES

Tofu "Fried" Rice

MAKES 1 SERVING

- 2 ounces extra firm tofu
- ¼ cup finely chopped broccoli
- ¼ cup thawed frozen shelled edamame
- ⅓ cup cooked brown rice
- 1 tablespoon chopped green onion (green parts only)
- ½ teaspoon low-sodium soy sauce
- ⅛ teaspoon garlic powder
- ⅛ teaspoon sesame oil

MICROWAVE DIRECTIONS

1 Press tofu between paper towels to remove excess water. Cut into ½-inch cubes.

2 Combine tofu, broccoli and edamame in large microwavable mug; mix well. Microwave on HIGH 1 minute.

3 Stir in rice, green onion, soy sauce, garlic powder and oil. Microwave 1 minute or until heated through. Stir well before serving.

Kale with Lemon and Garlic

MAKES 8 SERVINGS

2 bunches kale or
  Swiss chard
  (1 to 1¼ pounds)

1 tablespoon olive oil

1 clove garlic, minced

½ cup reduced-
  sodium chicken or
  vegetable broth

½ teaspoon salt
  (optional)

¼ teaspoon black
  pepper

1 lemon, cut into
  8 wedges

1 Trim any tough stems from kale. Stack and thinly slice leaves. Heat oil in large saucepan over medium heat. Add garlic; cook 2 minutes, stirring frequently. Add chopped kale and broth; cover and simmer 7 minutes. Stir kale; cover and simmer over medium-low heat 8 to 10 minutes or until kale is tender.

2 Stir in salt, if desired, and pepper. Squeeze wedge of lemon over each serving.

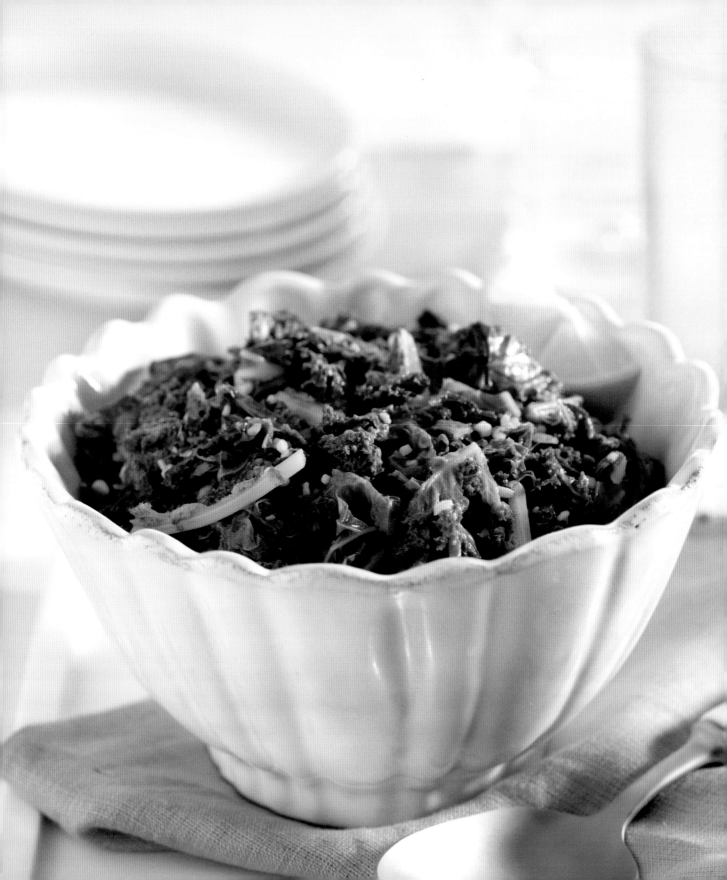

Wilted Spinach Salad with White Beans & Olives

MAKES 4 SERVINGS

1 tablespoon olive oil

¼ cup chopped onion

1 can (about 15 ounces) navy beans, rinsed and drained

½ cup halved pitted kalamata or black olives

1 package (9 ounces) baby spinach

¾ cup cherry tomatoes, halved

1½ tablespoons balsamic vinegar

Black pepper (optional)

1 Heat oil in large saucepan over medium heat. Add onion; cook, stirring occasionally, 5 to 6 minutes or until onion is tender. Stir in beans and olives; heat through.

2 Add spinach, tomatoes and vinegar; cover and cook 1 minute or until spinach is slightly wilted. Turn off heat; toss lightly. Transfer to serving plates. Season with pepper, if desired.

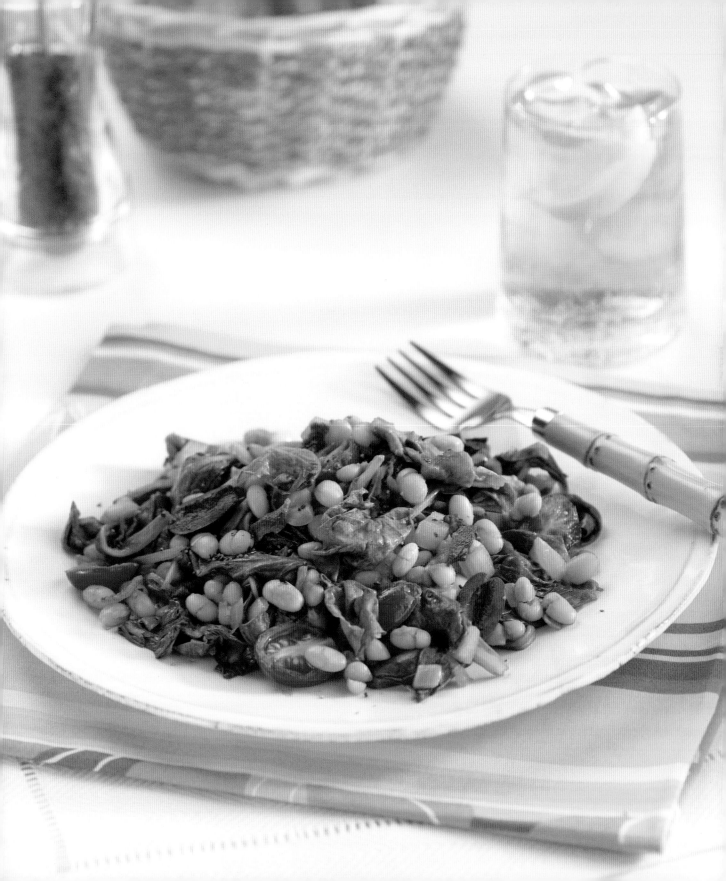

Chilled Cucumber Soup

MAKES 4 SERVINGS

1 large cucumber, peeled and coarsely chopped

6 ounces plain nonfat Greek yogurt

¼ cup packed fresh dill

½ teaspoon salt (optional)

⅛ teaspoon white pepper (optional)

1½ cups fat-free reduced-sodium chicken or vegetable broth

Sprigs fresh dill (optional)

1 Place cucumber in food processor; process until finely chopped. Add yogurt, ¼ cup dill, salt and white pepper, if desired; process until fairly smooth.

2 Transfer mixture to large bowl; stir in broth. Cover and chill at least 2 hours or up to 24 hours. Ladle into shallow bowls; garnish with dill sprigs.

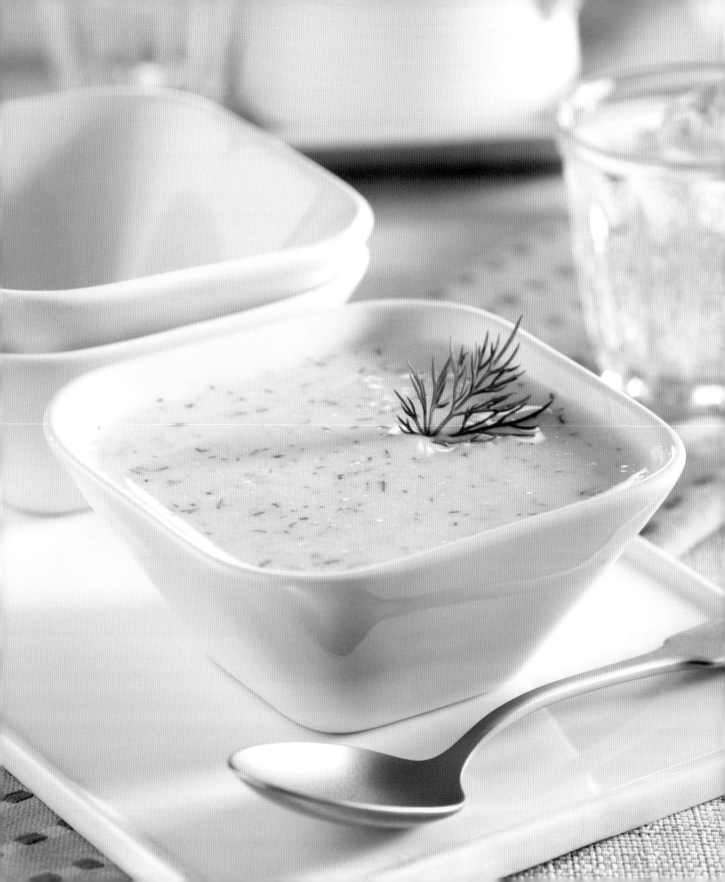

Acorn Squash Soup with Chicken and Red Pepper Meatballs

MAKES 2 SERVINGS

1 small to medium acorn squash (about ¾ pound)

½ pound ground lean chicken or turkey

1 red bell pepper, seeded and finely chopped

3 tablespoons cholesterol-free egg substitute

1 teaspoon dried parsley flakes

1 teaspoon ground coriander

½ teaspoon black pepper

¼ teaspoon ground cinnamon

3 cups reduced-sodium vegetable broth

2 tablespoons plain nonfat Greek yogurt (optional)

Ground red pepper (optional)

1 Pierce squash skin with fork. Place in microwaveable dish; microwave on HIGH 8 to 10 minutes or until tender. Cool 10 minutes.

2 Meanwhile, combine chicken, bell pepper, egg substitute, parsley flakes, coriander, black pepper and cinnamon in large bowl, mix lightly. Shape mixture into 8 meatballs. Place meatballs in microwavable dish; microwave on HIGH 5 minutes or until cooked through. Set aside to cool.

3 Remove and discard seeds from cooled squash. Scrape squash flesh from shell into large saucepan; mash squash with potato masher. Add broth and meatballs to saucepan; cook over medium-high heat 12 minutes, stirring occasionally. Add additional liquid, if necessary.

4 Garnish each serving with 1 tablespoon yogurt and ground red pepper, if desired.

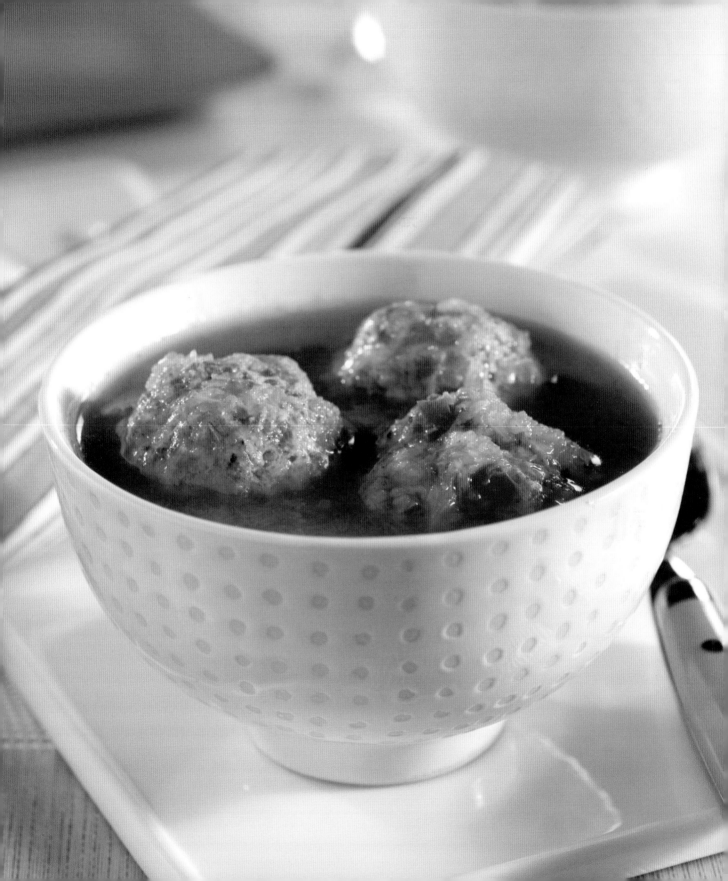

Mediterranean Stew

MAKES 6 SERVINGS

1 medium butternut or acorn squash, peeled and cut into 1-inch cubes

2 cups unpeeled eggplant, cut into 1-inch cubes

2 cups sliced zucchini

1 can (about 15 ounces) chickpeas, rinsed and drained

1 package (10 ounces) frozen cut okra

1 can (8 ounces) tomato sauce

¼ cup chopped onion

1 medium tomato, chopped

1 medium carrot, thinly sliced

½ cup reduced-sodium vegetable broth

¼ cup raisins

½ teaspoon ground cumin

½ teaspoon ground turmeric

¼ to ½ teaspoon ground red pepper

¼ teaspoon ground cinnamon

¼ teaspoon paprika

6 cups hot cooked couscous or brown rice

Fresh chopped parsley (optional)

SLOW COOKER DIRECTIONS

1 Combine squash, eggplant, zucchini, chickpeas, okra, tomato sauce, onion, tomato, carrot, broth, raisins, cumin, turmeric, ground red pepper, cinnamon and paprika in slow cooker; mix well. Cover; cook on LOW 8 to 10 hours or until vegetables are crisp-tender.

2 Serve over couscous. Garnish with parsley.

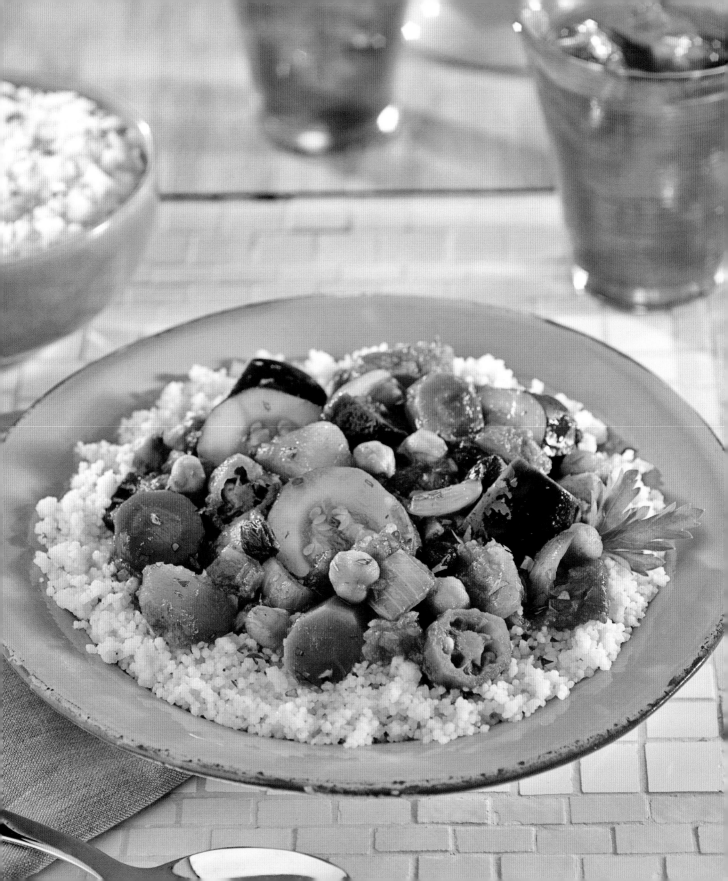

Couscous and Black Bean Salad

MAKES 4 SERVINGS

- 1⅓ cups cooked whole wheat couscous
- 1 can (about 15 ounces) black beans, rinsed and drained
- ½ cup cherry tomatoes,
- 2 tablespoons minced fresh chives or green onion (green parts only)
- 1 tablespoon minced fresh cilantro
- 1 small jalapeño pepper,* cored, seeded and minced (optional)
- 2 teaspoons white wine vinegar
- 1 teaspoon olive oil
- ¼ teaspoon salt
- ⅛ teaspoon black pepper

*Jalapeño peppers can sting and irritate the skin, so wear rubber gloves when handling peppers and do not touch your eyes.

1 Combine couscous and black beans in large bowl. Cut tomatoes in half lengthwise. Add tomatoes to couscous. Stir in chives, cilantro and jalapeño pepper, if desired; mix gently.

2 Whisk vinegar, oil, salt and black pepper in small bowl until well blended. Pour over salad; toss lightly to coat.

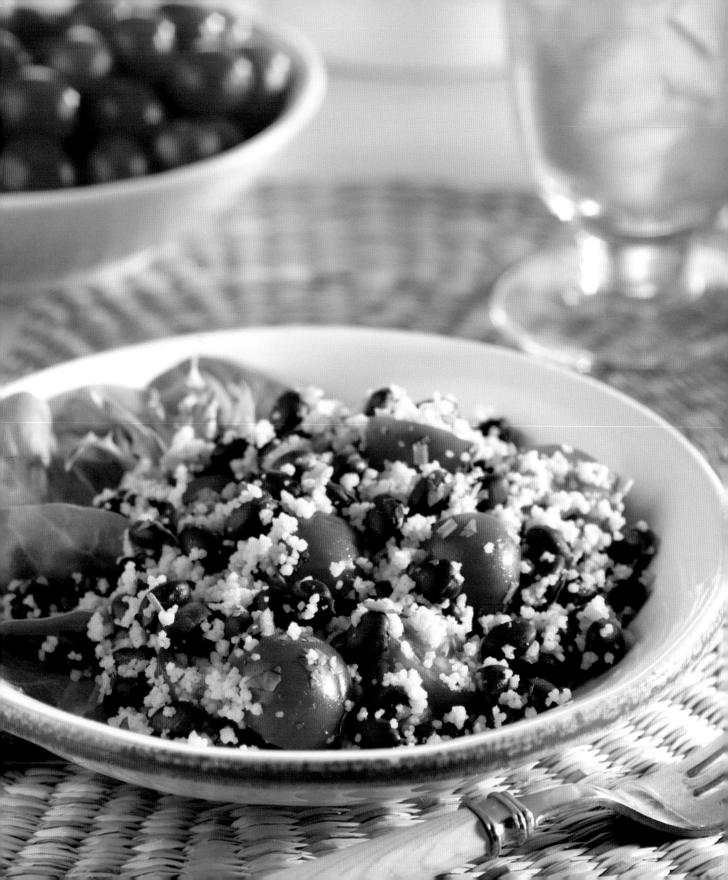

Cucumber-Jicama Salad

MAKES 6 SERVINGS

- 1 **cucumber, unpeeled**
- 1 **jicama (1¼ to 1½ pounds)**
- ¼ **cup thinly slivered mild red onion (optional)**
- 2 **tablespoons fresh lime juice**
- ½ **teaspoon grated lime peel**
- ¼ **teaspoon salt**
- ⅛ **teaspoon crumbled dried de árbol chile or red pepper flakes**
- 3 **tablespoons vegetable oil**
  - **Leaf lettuce**
  - **Lime wedges (optional)**

1 Cut cucumber lengthwise in half; scoop out and discard seeds. Cut halves crosswise into ⅛-inch-thick slices. Peel jicama. Cut lengthwise into 8 wedges; cut wedges crosswise into ⅛-inch-thick slices.

2 Combine cucumber, jicama and onion, if desired, in large bowl; toss lightly to mix; set aside.

3 Combine juice, lime peel, salt and chile in small bowl. Gradually add oil, whisking continuously, until dressing is thoroughly blended.

4 Pour dressing over salad; toss lightly to coat. Cover; refrigerate 1 to 2 hours to blend flavors.

5 Serve salad in lettuce-lined salad bowl. Garnish with lime wedges, if desired.

TIP

To add a decorative touch to cucumber slices, score the skin of a cucumber by pulling the tines of a dinner fork along the length of the cucumber. Rotate the cucumber and repeat until completely scored. Then cut the cucumber crosswise into slices.

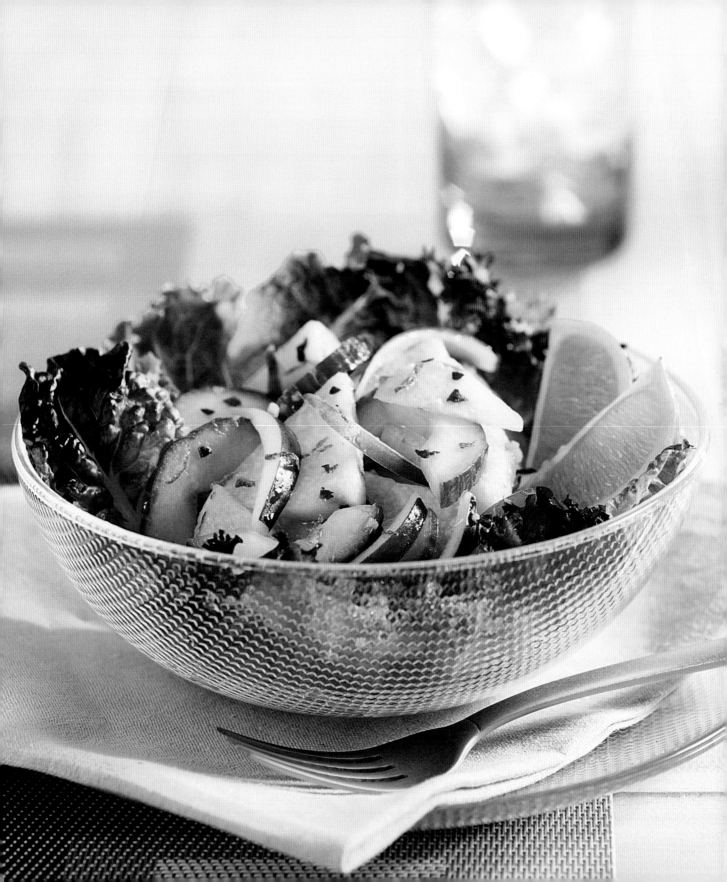

Spinach-Pine Nut Whole Grain Pilaf

MAKES 6 SERVINGS

2 cups hot cooked brown rice

1½ ounces pine nuts or slivered almonds, toasted

2 ounces spinach leaves, coarsely chopped

1 tablespoon extra virgin olive oil

1 teaspoon dried basil

½ teaspoon salt

¼ teaspoon red pepper flakes

Place hot rice in large bowl. Add remaining ingredients and toss gently, yet thoroughly until spinach is slightly wilted.

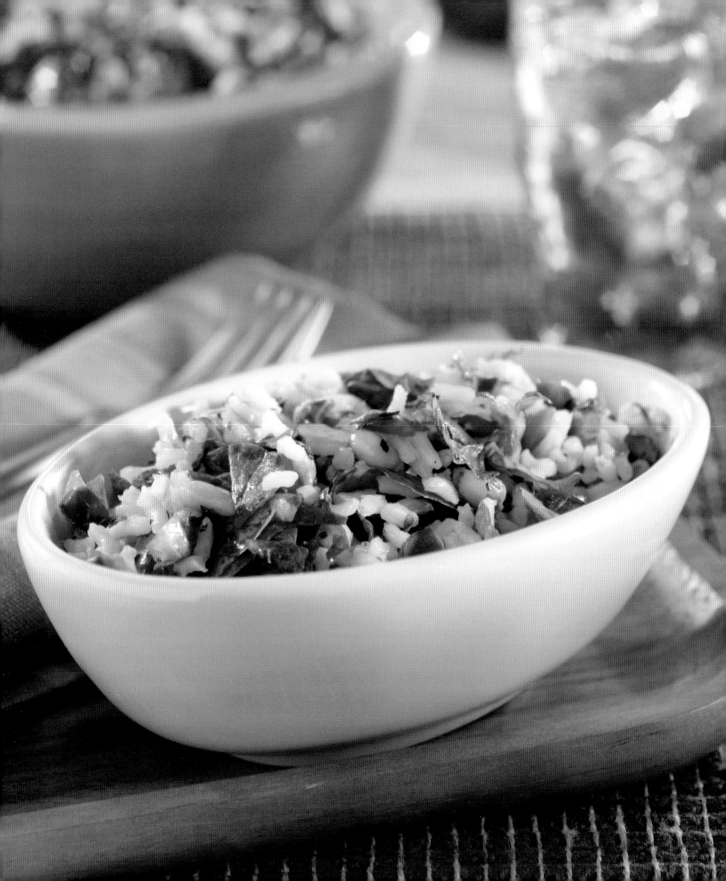

Favorite Green Beans

MAKES 6 SERVINGS

1 pound green beans
2 tablespoons olive oil
¼ cup grated Parmesan cheese
½ teaspoon garlic powder

1 Bring 1 quart of water to a boil in large saucepan. Add green beans and boil 3 minutes. Remove from heat and drain.

2 Heat oil in large skillet over medium heat. Add green beans to skillet. Cook 5 minutes, stirring occasionally. Remove from heat; sprinkle with Parmesan cheese and garlic powder. Serve warm.

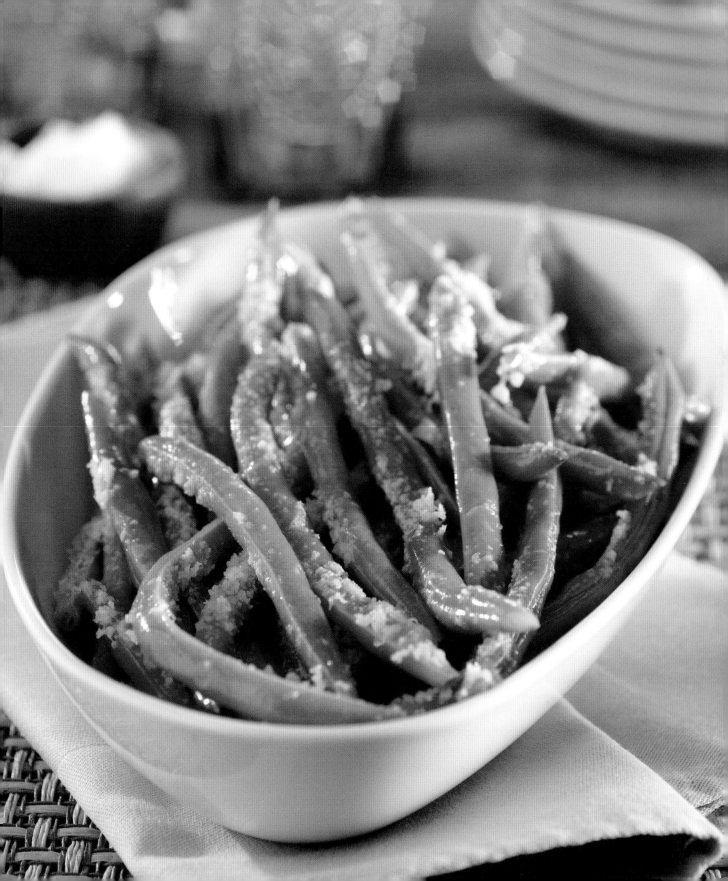

Mashed Sweet Potatoes & Parsnips

MAKES 6 SERVINGS

2 large sweet potatoes (about 1¼ pounds), peeled and cut into 1-inch pieces

2 medium parsnips (about ½ pound), peeled and cut into ½-inch slices

¼ cup unsweetened canned coconut milk

1 tablespoon butter

½ teaspoon salt

⅛ teaspoon ground nutmeg

¼ cup chopped fresh chives

1 Combine sweet potatoes and parsnips in large saucepan. Cover with cold water; bring to a boil over high heat. Reduce heat; simmer, uncovered, 15 minutes or until vegetables are tender.

2 Drain vegetables; return to pan. Add milk, butter, salt and nutmeg. Mash with potato masher over low heat until desired consistency is reached. Stir in chives.

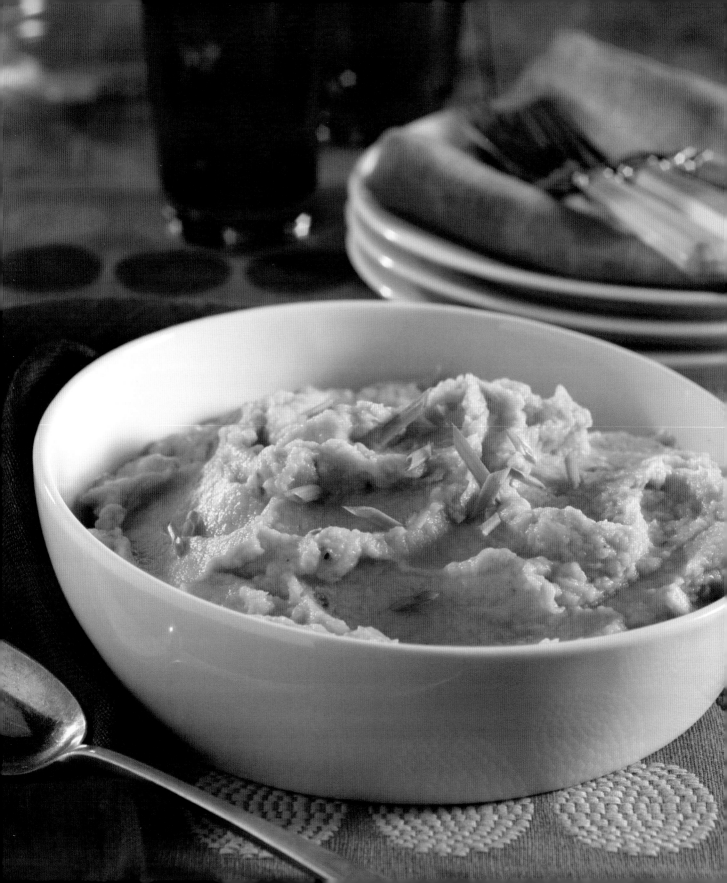

Pepper and Squash Gratin

MAKES 8 SERVINGS

1 russet potato
(12 ounces),
unpeeled

8 ounces yellow
summer squash,
thinly sliced

8 ounces zucchini,
thinly sliced

2 cups frozen bell
pepper stir-fry
blend, thawed

1 teaspoon dried
oregano

½ teaspoon salt

⅛ teaspoon black
pepper (optional)

½ cup grated
Parmesan cheese
or shredded
reduced-fat sharp
Cheddar cheese
(optional)

1 tablespoon olive oil

1 Preheat oven to 375°F. Spray 12×8-inch glass baking dish with nonstick cooking spray. Pierce potato several times with fork. Microwave on HIGH 3 minutes. Cut potato into thin slices.

2 Layer half of potato slices, yellow squash, zucchini, bell pepper blend, oregano, salt, black pepper and cheese, if desired, in prepared baking dish. Repeat layers. Drizzle with oil. Cover tightly with foil; bake 25 minutes or until vegetables are just tender. Remove foil; bake 10 minutes or until lightly browned.

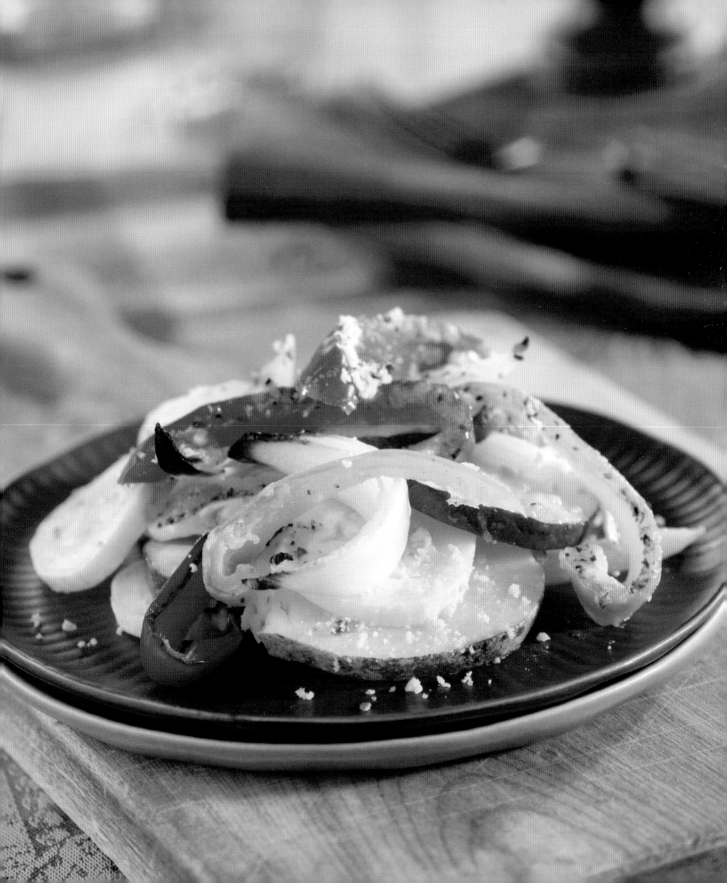

Heirloom Tomato Quinoa Salad

MAKES 4 SERVINGS

1 cup uncooked quinoa

2 cups water

2 tablespoons olive oil

1 tablespoon lemon juice

½ teaspoon garlic powder

½ teaspoon salt

1 cup assorted heirloom grape tomatoes (red, yellow or a combination), halved

¼ cup crumbled reduced-fat feta cheese (optional)

¼ cup chopped fresh basil, plus additional basil leaves for garnish

1 Place quinoa in fine-mesh strainer; rinse well under cold running water. Bring 2 cups water to a boil in small saucepan; stir in quinoa. Reduce heat to low; cover and simmer 10 to 15 minutes or until quinoa is tender and water is absorbed.

2 Meanwhile, whisk oil, lemon juice, garlic powder and salt in large bowl until well blended. Gently stir in tomatoes and quinoa. Cover and refrigerate at least 30 minutes.

3 Stir in cheese, if desired, just before serving. Top each serving with 1 tablespoon chopped basil. Garnish with additional basil leaves.

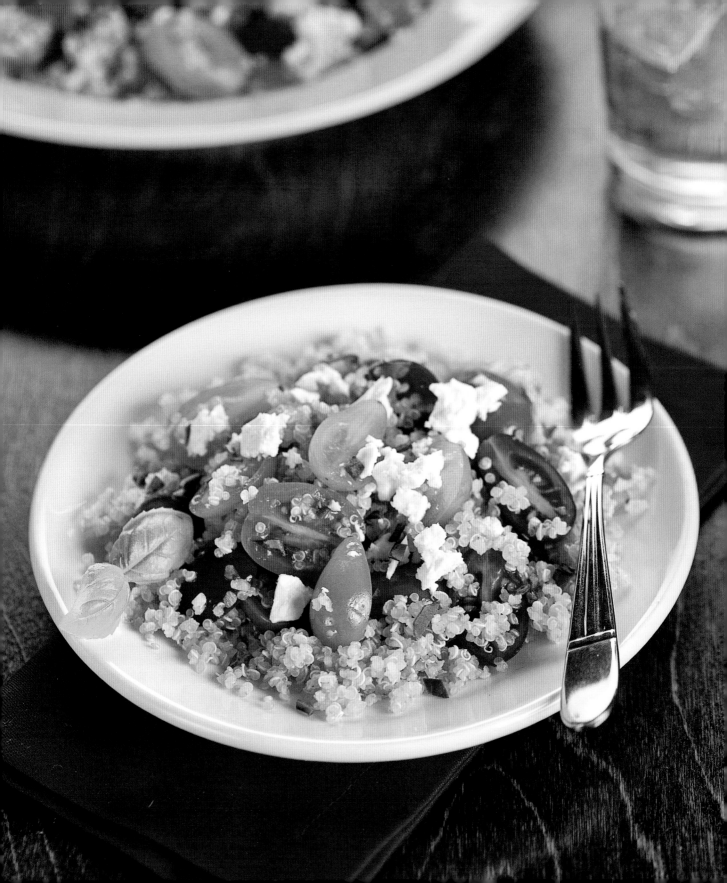

Tabbouleh-Style Amaranth Salad

MAKES 5 TO 6 SERVINGS

2½ cups water

¾ cup dried amaranth*

2 cups chopped fresh parsley

½ cup grape tomatoes, quartered

¼ cup diced red onion

3 tablespoons capers, drained (optional)

½ teaspoon garlic powder

1 ounce (¼ cup) pine nuts, toasted

2 tablespoons cider vinegar or red wine vinegar

1 tablespoon extra virgin olive oil

⅛ teaspoon red pepper flakes (optional)

¼ teaspoon salt

¾ cup (4 ounces) reduced-fat feta cheese, crumbled

Amaranth is an ancient whole grain and is very high in protein and fiber. In addition, it's gluten-free and a good source of iron and vitamin C. You can find it at the supermarket with the other grains or in bulk bins at health food stores.

1 Combine water and amaranth in large saucepan; bring to a boil over high heat. Reduce heat, cover and simmer 20 minutes or until most of the water is absorbed. (It will have a very soft consistency.)

2 Meanwhile, combine remaining ingredients except feta cheese, in medium bowl; set aside.

3 Place amaranth in fine-mesh strainer; rinse well under cold running water until completely cooled. Shake off excess liquid, add to parsley mixture; toss until well blended. Stir in feta; toss gently.

TIP

It's important that the amaranth is placed in a fine-mesh strainer. The grain is so tiny and will slip through a traditional strainer. Strain in 2 or 3 batches if using a small-mesh strainer.

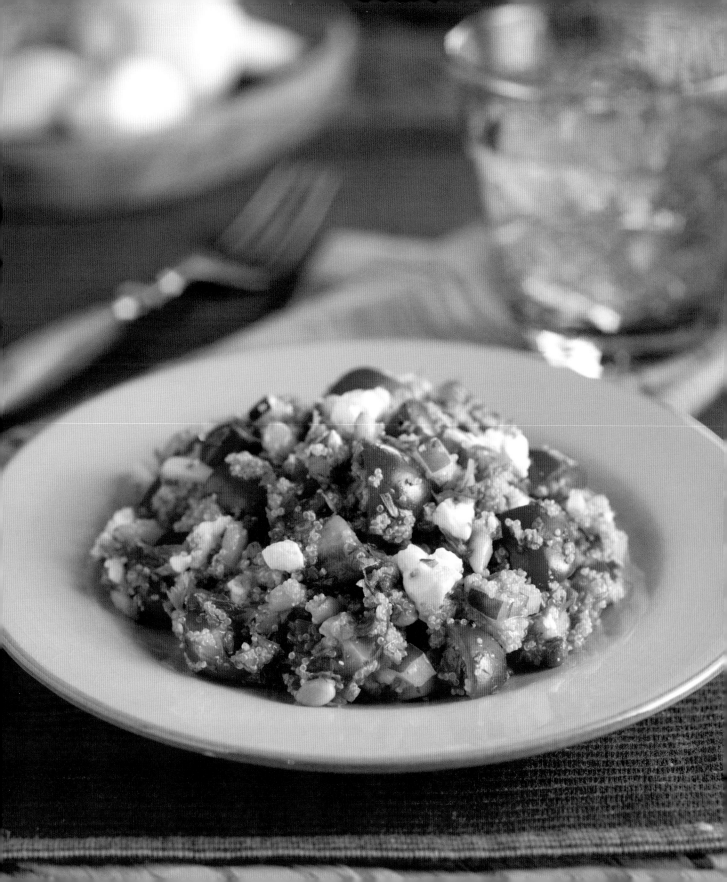

Roman Spinach Soup

MAKES 8 SERVINGS

6 cups fat-free reduced-sodium chicken broth

1 cup cholesterol-free egg substitute

¼ cup minced fresh basil

3 tablespoons grated Parmesan cheese

2 tablespoons fresh lemon juice

1 tablespoon minced fresh parsley

¼ teaspoon white pepper

⅛ teaspoon ground nutmeg

8 cups packed fresh spinach, chopped

Fresh lemon slices (optional)

1 Bring broth to a boil in 4-quart saucepan over medium heat.

2 Beat together egg substitute, basil, Parmesan cheese, lemon juice, parsley, white pepper and nutmeg in small bowl. Set aside.

3 Stir spinach into broth; simmer 1 minute. Slowly pour egg mixture into broth mixture, whisking constantly so egg threads form. Simmer 2 to 3 minutes or until egg is cooked. Garnish with lemon slices. Serve immediately.

NOTE

Soup may look curdled.

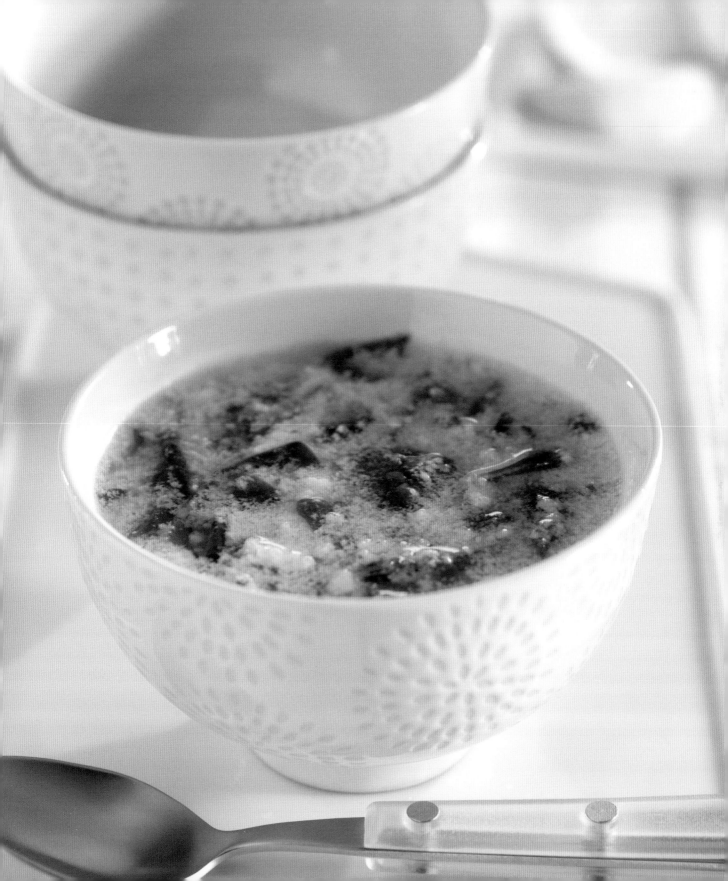

Spicy Sesame Noodles

MAKES 6 SERVINGS

6 ounces uncooked soba (buckwheat) noodles

2 teaspoons dark sesame oil

1 tablespoon sesame seeds

½ cup fat-free reduced-sodium chicken broth

1 tablespoon creamy peanut butter

¼ cup thinly sliced green onions (green parts only)

½ cup minced red bell pepper

4 teaspoons reduced-sodium soy sauce

1½ teaspoons finely chopped seeded jalapeño pepper*

¼ teaspoon red pepper flakes

Jalapeño peppers can sting and irritate the skin, so wear rubber gloves when handling peppers and do not touch your eyes.

1 Cook noodles according to package directions. (Do not overcook.) Rinse noodles thoroughly with cold running water; drain. Place noodles in large bowl; toss with oil.

2 Cook sesame seeds in small skillet over medium heat about 3 minutes or until seeds begin to pop and turn golden brown, stirring frequently. Remove from skillet.

3 Whisk broth and peanut butter in medium bowl until blended. (Mixture may look curdled.) Stir in green onions, bell pepper, soy sauce, jalapeño pepper and red pepper flakes.

4 Pour mixture over noodles; toss to coat. Cover and let stand 30 minutes at room temperature or refrigerate up to 24 hours. Sprinkle with toasted sesame seeds before serving.

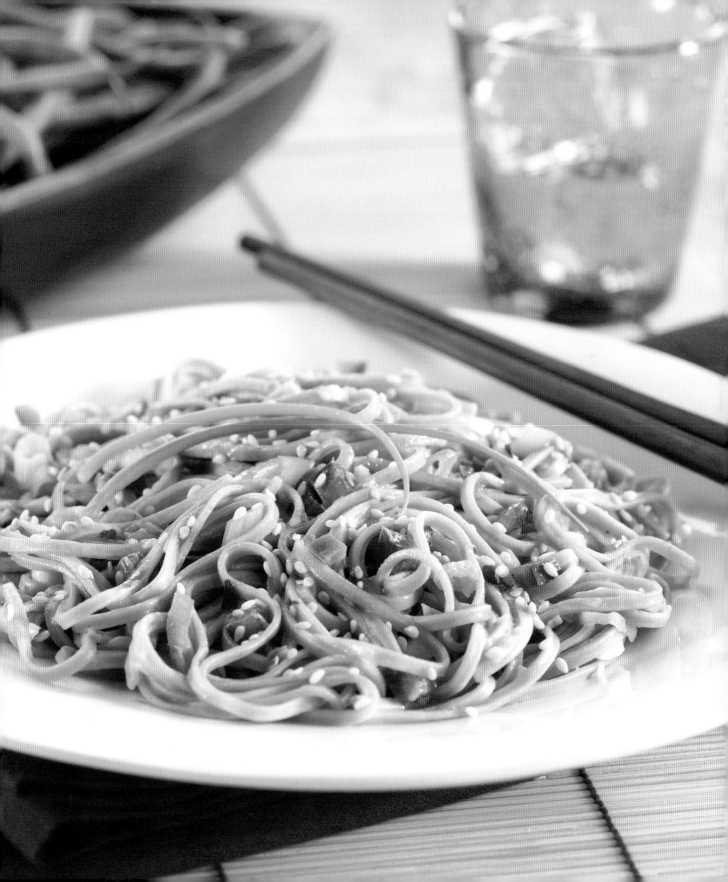

Italian Eggplant with Millet and Pepper Stuffing

MAKES 4 SERVINGS

¼ cup uncooked millet

2 small eggplants (about ¾ pound total)

¼ cup chopped red bell pepper, divided

¼ cup chopped green bell pepper, divided

1 teaspoon olive oil

1½ cups fat-free reduced-sodium vegetable broth

½ teaspoon ground cumin

½ teaspoon dried oregano

⅛ teaspoon red pepper flakes

1 Cook and stir millet in large heavy skillet over medium heat 5 minutes or until golden. Transfer to small bowl; set aside.

2 Slice eggplants in half lengthwise. Scoop out flesh, leaving ¼-inch shell. Finely chop scooped out flesh and set aside. Combine 1 tablespoon red bell pepper and 1 tablespoon green bell pepper in small bowl; set aside.

3 Heat oil in same skillet over medium heat. Add chopped eggplant and remaining red and green bell pepper; cook and stir about 8 minutes or until eggplant is tender.

4 Stir in toasted millet, broth, cumin, oregano and red pepper flakes. Bring to a boil over high heat. Reduce heat to medium-low. Cook, covered, 35 minutes or until all liquid has been absorbed and millet is tender. Remove from heat; let stand, covered, 10 minutes.

5 Preheat oven to 350°F. Pour 1 cup water into 8-inch square baking pan. Fill eggplant shells with eggplant-millet mixture. Sprinkle with reserved chopped bell peppers, pressing in lightly. Carefully place filled shells in prepared pan. Bake 15 minutes or until heated through.

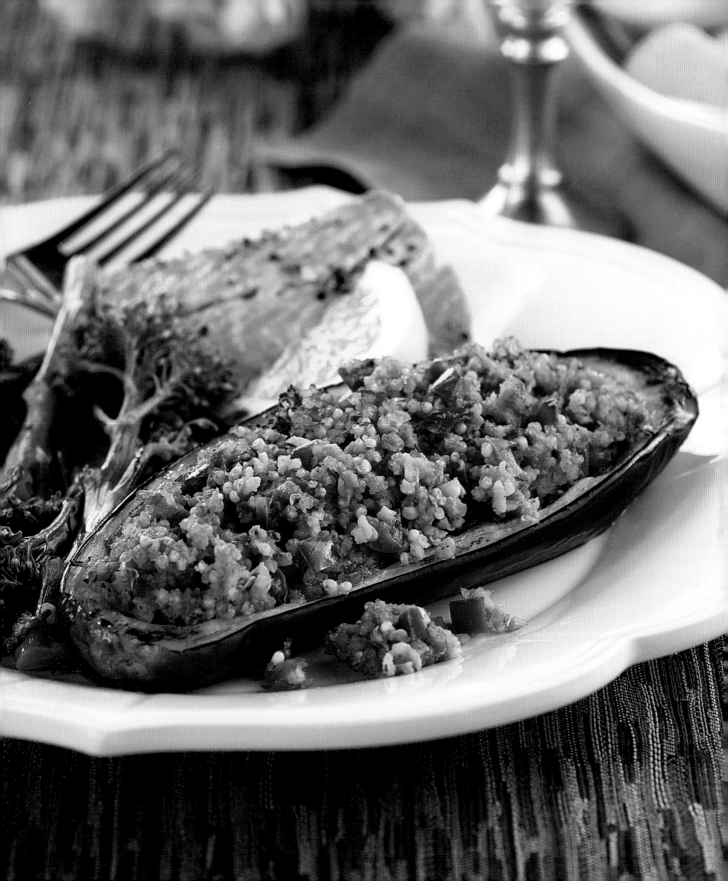

Quinoa & Vegetable Medley

MAKES 6 SERVINGS

2 medium sweet potatoes, cut into ½-inch-thick slices

1 medium eggplant, peeled and cut into ½-inch cubes

1 medium tomato, cut into wedges

1 large green bell pepper, sliced

1 small onion, cut into wedges

½ teaspoon salt

¼ teaspoon black pepper

¼ teaspoon ground red pepper

1 cup uncooked quinoa

½ teaspoon dried thyme

¼ teaspoon dried marjoram

2 cups water or fat-free reduced-sodium vegetable broth

SLOW COOKER DIRECTIONS

1 Coat slow cooker with nonstick cooking spray. Combine sweet potatoes, eggplant, tomato, bell pepper, onion, salt, black pepper and ground red pepper in slow cooker; toss to coat.

2 Meanwhile, place quinoa in fine-mesh strainer; rinse well under cold running water. Add to vegetable mixture. Stir in thyme, marjoram and broth. Cover; cook on LOW 5 hours or on HIGH 2½ hours until quinoa is tender and broth is absorbed.

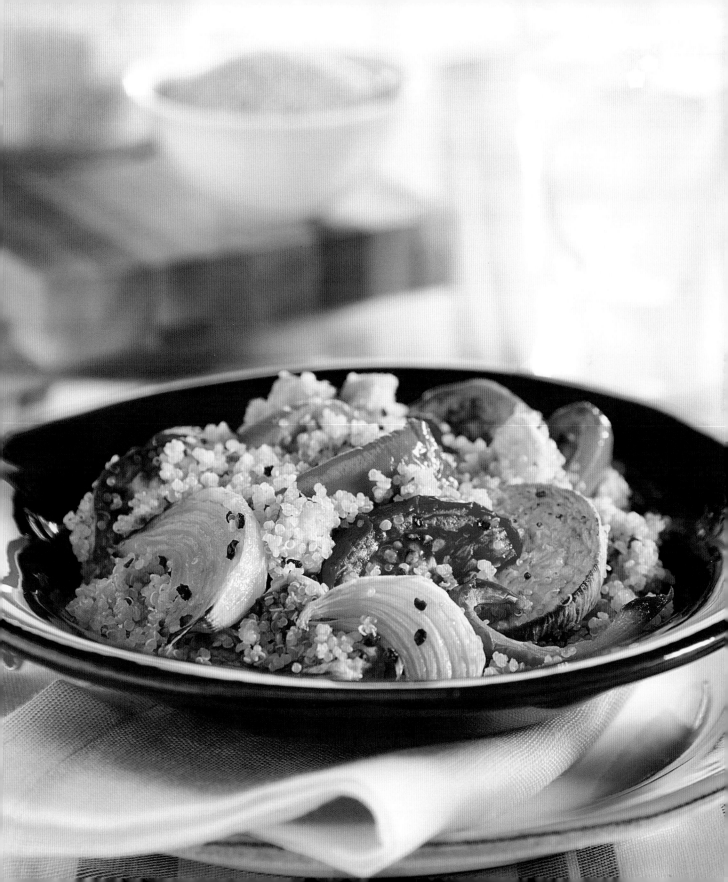

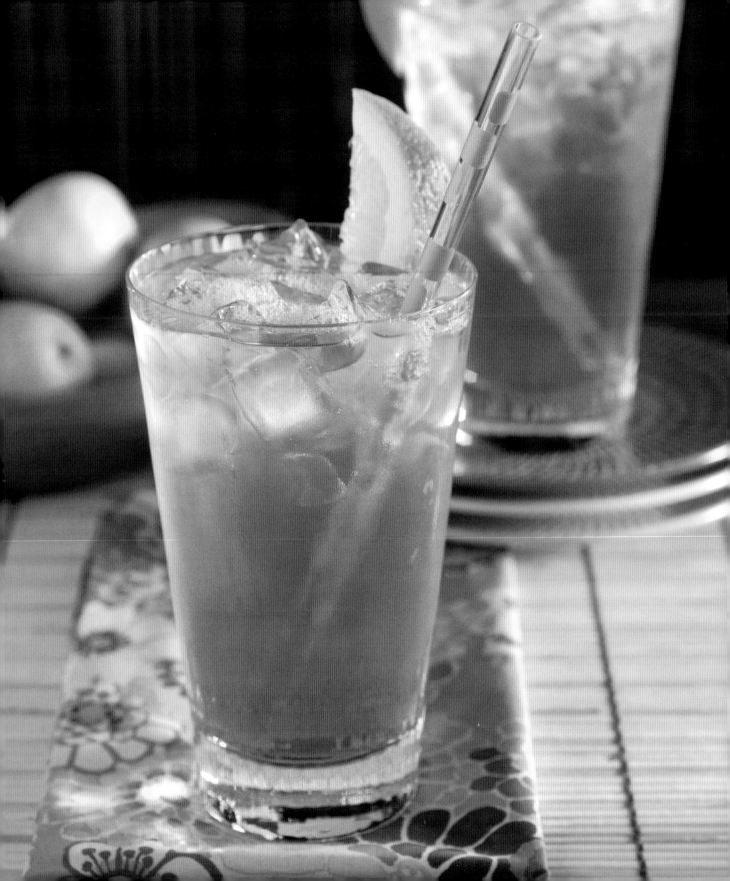

BEVERAGES & SMOOTHIES

Orange Tea Zinger

MAKES 2 SERVINGS

2 orange or tangerine-
  flavored herbal tea
  bags

1 cup boiling water

  Ice

2 cans (12 ounces
  each) unsweetened
  seltzer water

1 Steep both tea bags in boiling water for about 4 minutes to brew 1 cup of double-strength tea. Remove tea bags and refrigerate until cool.

2 To serve, pour half of cooled tea (just less than ½ cup) over ice in each of 2 tall glasses. Fill glasses with seltzer water and stir gently.

Go Green Smoothie

MAKES 1 SERVING

1½ cups ice cubes

1 cup packed torn spinach

½ cup vanilla almond milk

¼ cup vanilla low-fat yogurt

¼ avocado

1 teaspoon lemon juice

Combine ice, spinach, milk, yogurt, avocado and lemon juice in blender; blend until smooth.

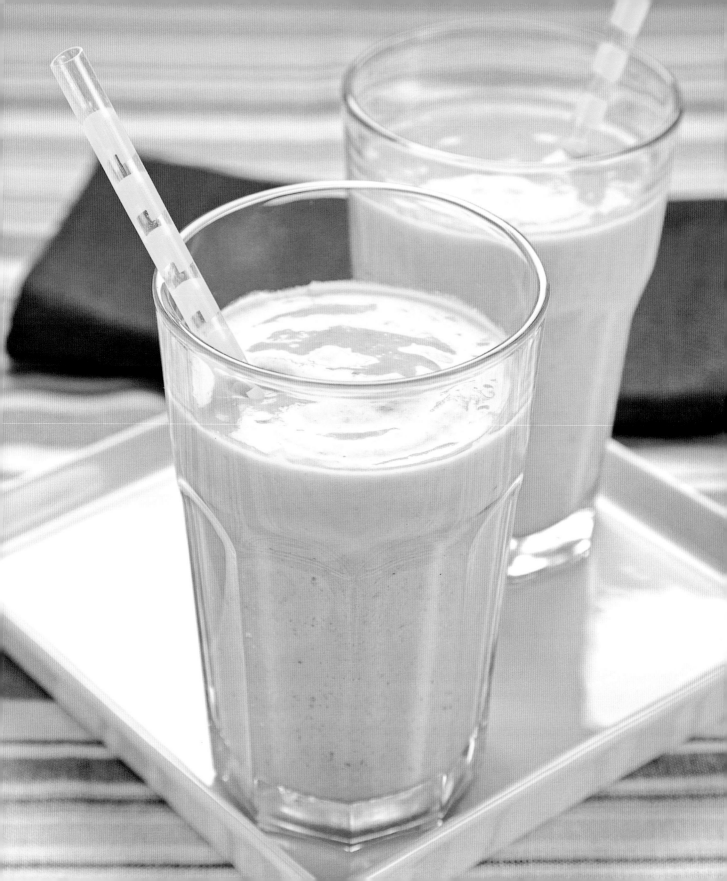

Cool Cucumber

MAKES 2 SERVINGS

1 **cucumber**
¼ **pineapple, peeled**
¼ **cup fresh cilantro**

Juice cucumber, pineapple and cilantro. Stir.

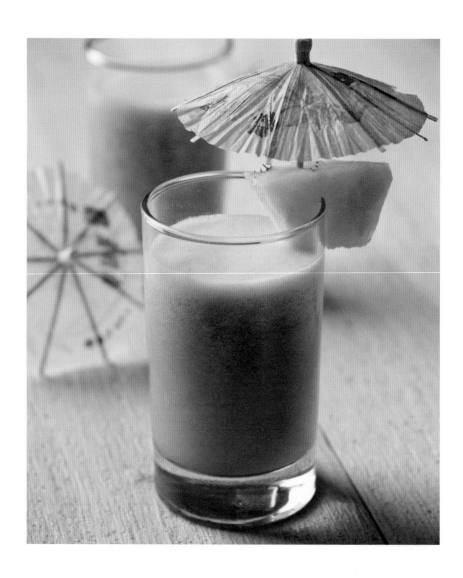

Bedtime Cocktail

MAKES 2 SERVINGS

½ **head romaine lettuce**
2 **stalks celery**
½ **cucumber**

Juice romaine, celery and cucumber. Stir.

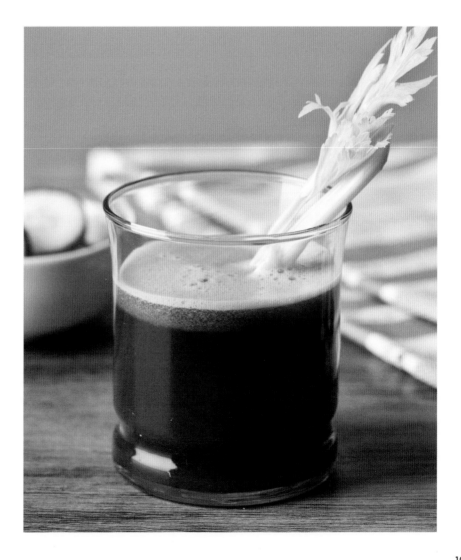

Fiery Cucumber Beet Juice

MAKES 2 SERVINGS

1   **cucumber**
1   **beet**
1   **lemon, peeled**
1   **inch fresh ginger, peeled**
½   **jalapeño pepper***

*Jalapeño peppers can sting and irritate the skin, so wear rubber gloves when handling peppers and do not touch your eyes.

Juice cucumber, beet, lemon, ginger and jalapeño pepper. Stir.

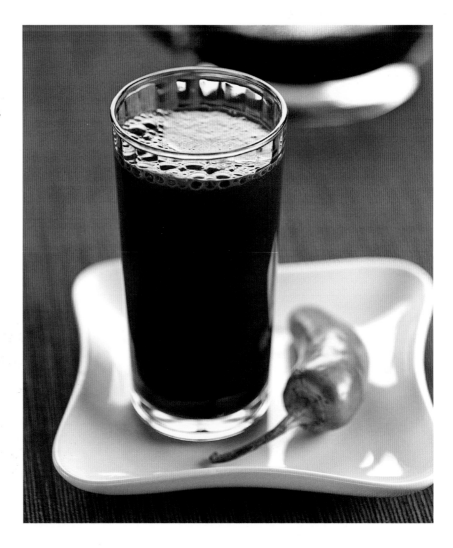

Spiced Pumpkin Banana Smoothie

MAKES 1 SERVING

- ½ **cup almond milk**
- ½ **frozen banana**
- ½ **cup unsweetened canned pumpkin**
- ½ **cup ice cubes**
- 1 **teaspoon ground flaxseeds**
- ¼ **teaspoon ground cinnamon**
- ⅛ **teaspoon ground ginger**
- **Dash ground nutmeg**

Combine almond milk, banana, pumpkin, ice, flaxseeds, cinnamon, ginger and nutmeg in blender; blend until smooth. Serve immediately.

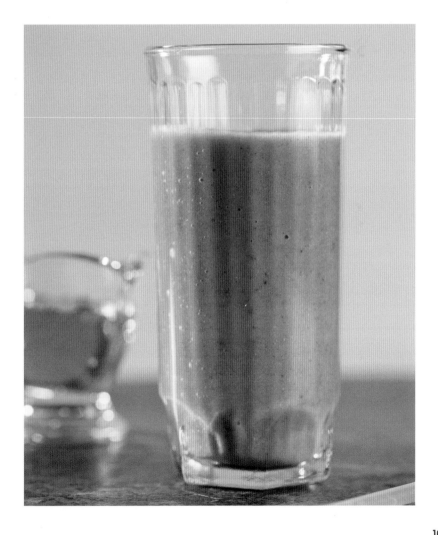

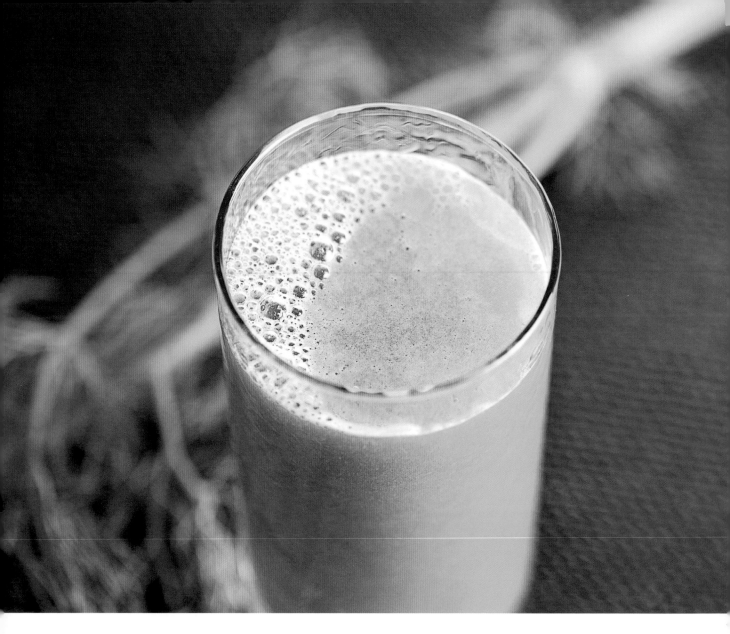

Cleansing Green Juice

MAKES 2 SERVINGS

 4 **leaves bok choy**
 1 **stalk celery**
 ½ **cucumber**
 ¼ **bulb fennel**
 ½ **lemon, peeled**

Juice bok choy, celery, cucumber, fennel and lemon. Stir.

Double Green Pineapple

MAKES 1 SERVING

4   leaves Swiss chard
4   leaves kale
¼   pineapple, peeled

Juice chard, kale and pineapple. Stir.

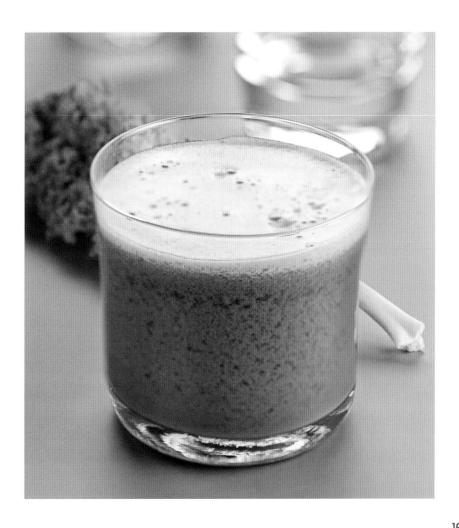

Ginger-Lime Iced Green Tea

MAKES 4 SERVINGS

1 quart water

2 thin slices fresh ginger (about 1 inch in diameter)

4 green tea bags

¼ cup freshly squeezed lime juice (2 to 3 limes)

Ice cubes

Lime slices (optional)

1 Bring water and ginger to a boil in large saucepan. Pour water over tea bags in teapot or 4-cup heatproof measuring cup; steep 3 minutes. Remove and discard tea bags and ginger. Cool tea to room temperature.

2 Add lime juice to tea. Pour tea into 4 ice-filled glasses. Sweeten with sugar substitute, such as stevia, if desired. Garnish with lime slices.

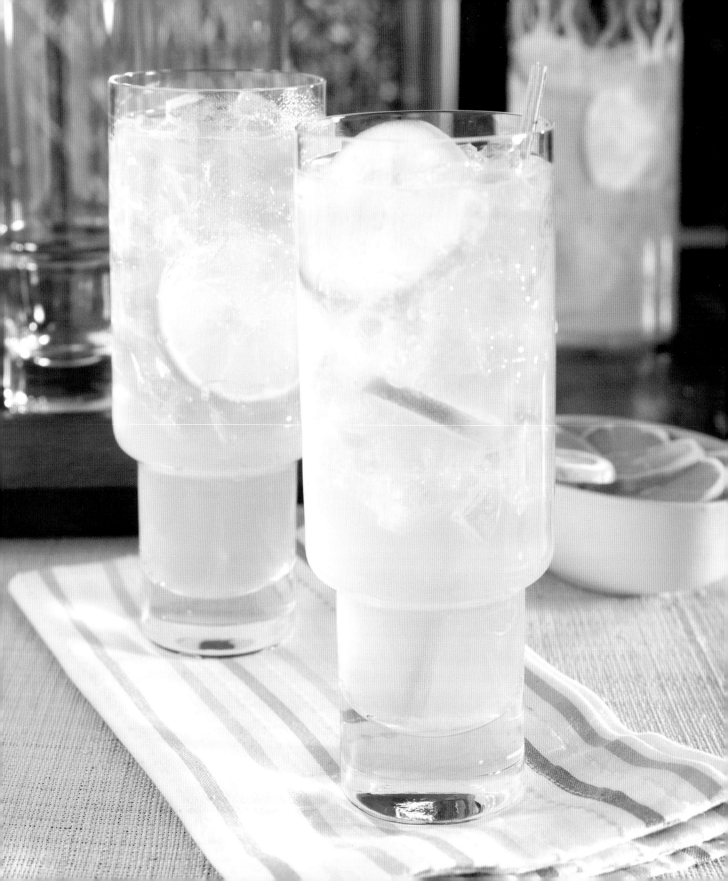

Cucumber Punch

MAKES 10 TO 12 SERVINGS

1 **English cucumber, thinly sliced**

1 **cup water**

4 **ounces thawed frozen limeade concentrate**

1 **bottle (1 liter) club soda, chilled**

Ice cubes

Lime wedges (optional)

1 Combine cucumber slices, water and limeade concentrate in punch bowl or pitcher. Refrigerate 1 hour.

2 Add club soda and ice just before serving. Pour into 10 glasses. Garnish with lime wedges.

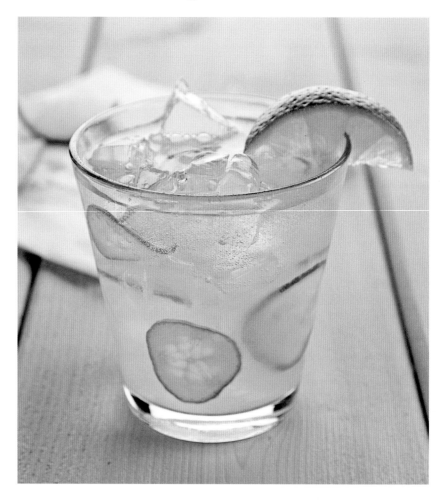

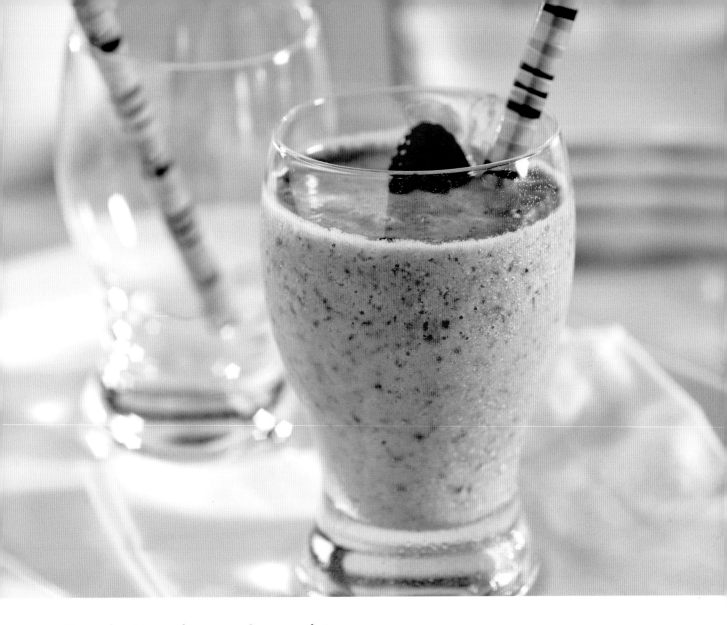

Simple Raspberry Smoothie

MAKES 2 SERVINGS

½ cup unsweetened
    coconut milk

1 cup fresh raspberries

½ cup ice cubes

Combine coconut milk, raspberries and ice in blender; blend until smooth. Serve immediately.

Chocolate Blueberry Shake

MAKES 1 SERVING

¼ **cup unsweetened almond milk**

½ **cup fresh blueberries**

¼ **cup ice cubes**

½ **teaspoon unsweetened cocoa powder**

Combine milk, blueberries, ice and cocoa in blender; blend until smooth. Serve immediately.

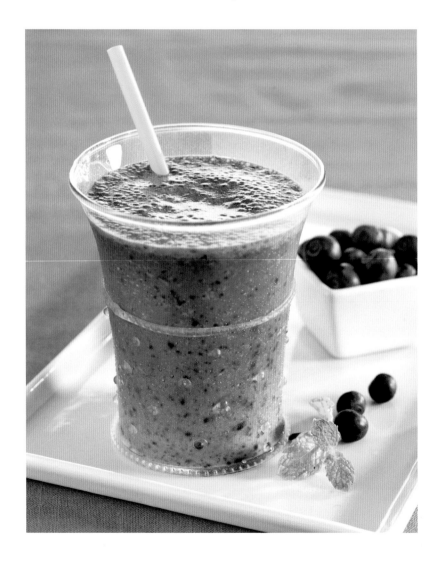

Blue Kale Smoothie

MAKES 2 SERVINGS

¼ **cup unsweetened almond milk**

1 **frozen banana**

1 **cup chopped fresh kale**

¼ **cup fresh blueberries**

¼ **cup ice cubes**

Combine milk, banana, kale, blueberries and ice in blender; blend until smooth. Serve immediately.

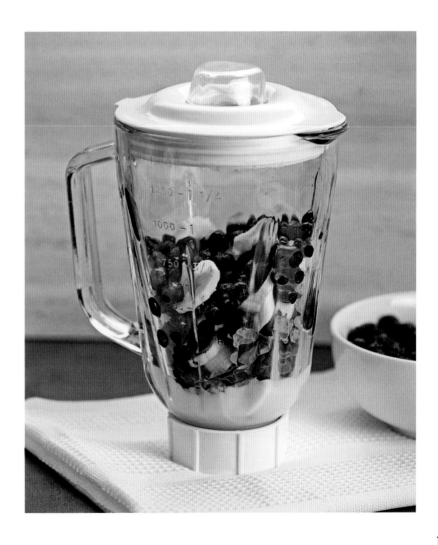

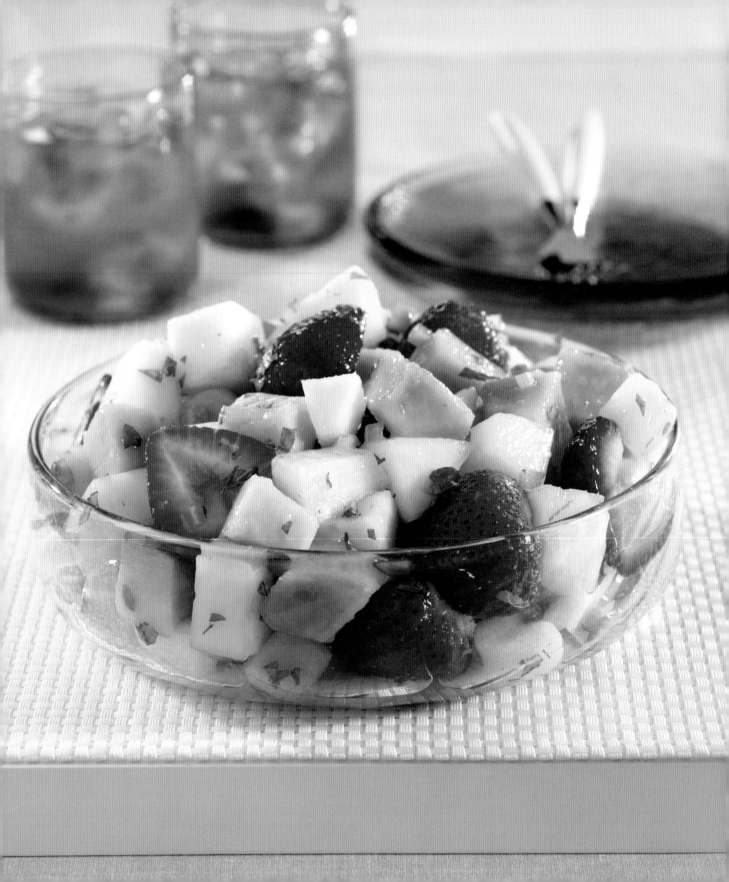

SNACKS & SWEETS

Hot and Spicy Fruit Salad

MAKES 8 SERVINGS

⅓ cup orange juice

3 tablespoons lime juice

3 tablespoons minced fresh mint, basil or cilantro, plus additional for garnish

2 jalapeño peppers,* seeded and minced

½ small honeydew melon, cut into cubes

1 pint fresh strawberries, stemmed, halved

1 cup fresh pineapple cubes

Jalapeño peppers can sting and irritate the skin, so wear rubber gloves when handling peppers and do not touch your eyes.

1 Blend orange juice, lime juice, 3 tablespoons mint and jalapeño peppers in small bowl.

2 Combine melon, strawberries and pineapple in large bowl. Pour orange juice mixture over fruit; toss gently until well blended.

3 Serve immediately or cover and refrigerate up to 3 hours. Garnish with fresh mint, if desired.

Toasted Coconut & Quinoa Balls

MAKES 24 SERVINGS

½ cup uncooked quinoa

1 cup water

2 cups sweetened flaked coconut (about ½ of 14-ounce package), divided

½ cup creamy almond butter

1 tablespoon maple syrup

½ teaspoon ground cinnamon

½ teaspoon vanilla

1 Preheat oven to 350°F. Place quinoa in fine-mesh strainer; rinse well under cold running water.

2 Bring 1 cup water and quinoa in medium saucepan to a boil over high heat. Reduce heat to low; cover and simmer 10 to 15 minutes or until quinoa is tender and water is absorbed. Cool slightly.

3 Meanwhile, spread coconut in shallow baking pan. Bake 7 to 10 minutes or until lightly brown and toasted, stirring frequently. Cool slightly.

4 Combine quinoa, 1¼ cups coconut, almond butter, maple syrup, cinnamon and vanilla in medium bowl.

5 Shape mixture into 1-inch balls. Roll in remaining ¾ cup coconut to coat. Store leftovers in refrigerator.

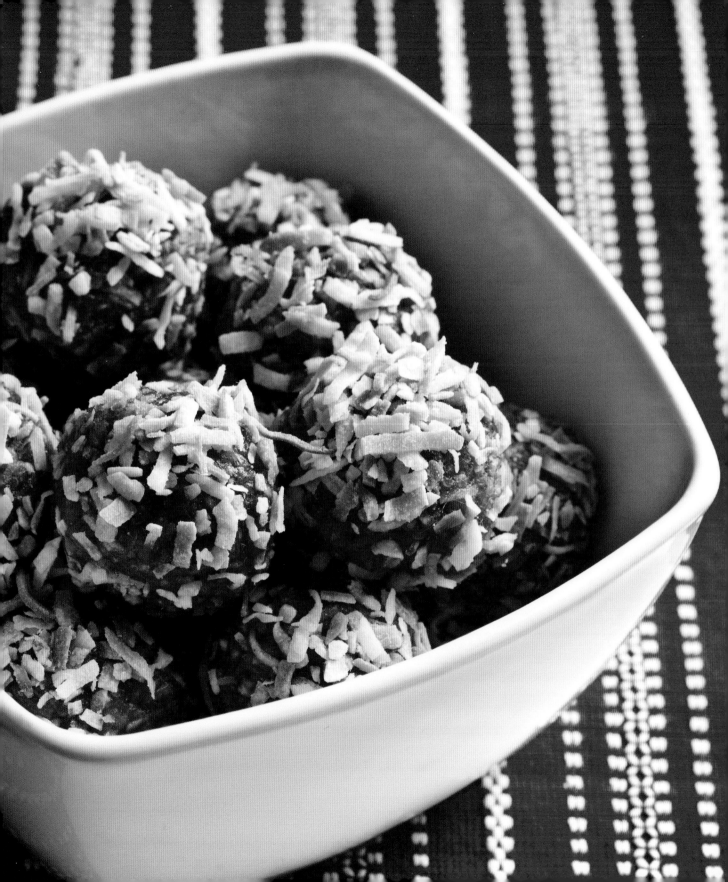

Kiwi & Strawberries with Pine Nuts

MAKES 4 SERVINGS

2 **kiwi fruits**

1½ **cups fresh strawberries**

1 **tablespoon orange juice**

1 **tablespoon pine nuts, toasted**

1 Peel kiwis and slice into thin rounds. Arrange on 4 dessert plates.

2 Wash, hull and slice strawberries. Arrange over kiwi slices. Drizzle orange juice evenly over each dish. Top evenly with pine nuts.

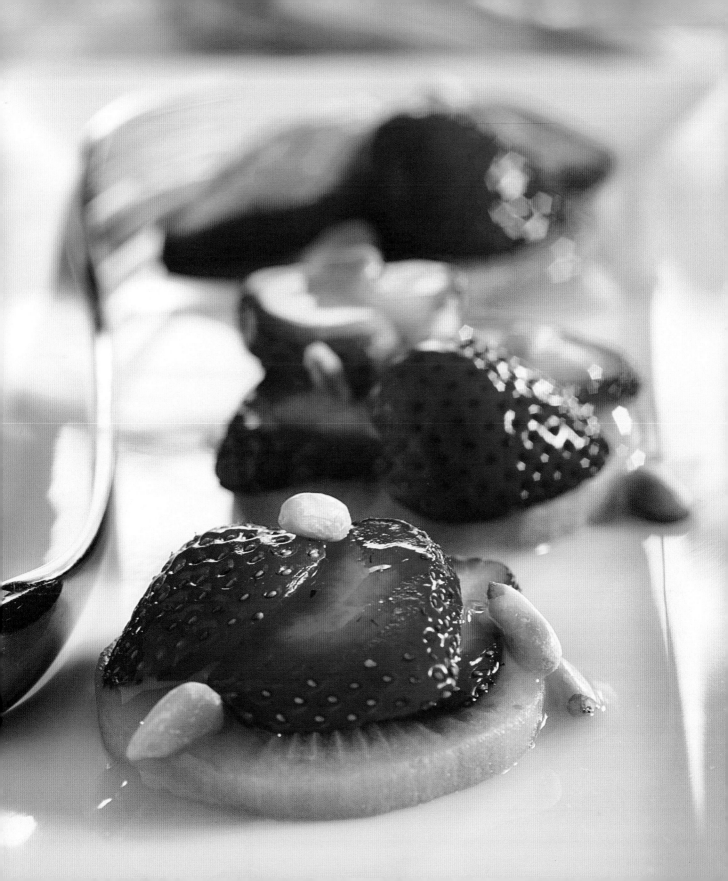

Spicy Roasted Chickpeas

MAKES 4 SERVINGS

1 can (about 15 ounces)
  chickpeas, rinsed
  and drained

3 tablespoons olive oil

½ teaspoon salt

½ teaspoon black
  pepper

¾ to 1 tablespoon chili
  powder

⅛ to ¼ teaspoon
  ground red pepper

1 lime, cut into
  wedges

1 Preheat oven to 400°F.

2 Combine chickpeas, oil, salt and black pepper in large bowl;
  toss to coat. Spread in single layer on 15×10-inch jelly-roll
  pan.

3 Bake 15 minutes or until chickpeas begin to brown, shaking
  pan twice.

4 Sprinkle with chili powder and ground red pepper. Bake
  5 minutes or until dark golden-red. Serve with lime wedges.

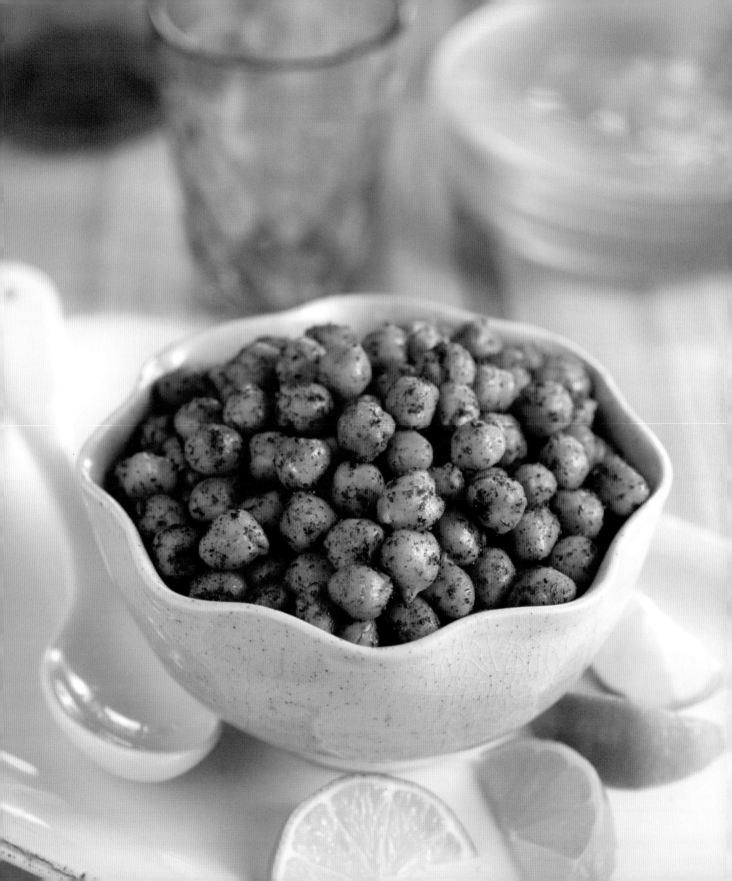

Fruit Kabobs with Raspberry Yogurt Dip

MAKES 6 SERVINGS

½ cup plain nonfat Greek yogurt

¼ cup no-sugar-added raspberry fruit spread

1 pint fresh strawberries

2 cups cubed honeydew melon (1-inch cubes)

2 cups cubed cantaloupe (1-inch cubes)

1 cup fresh pineapple cubes

1 Stir yogurt and fruit spread in small bowl until well blended.

2 Thread fruit alternately onto 6 (12-inch) skewers. Serve with yogurt dip.

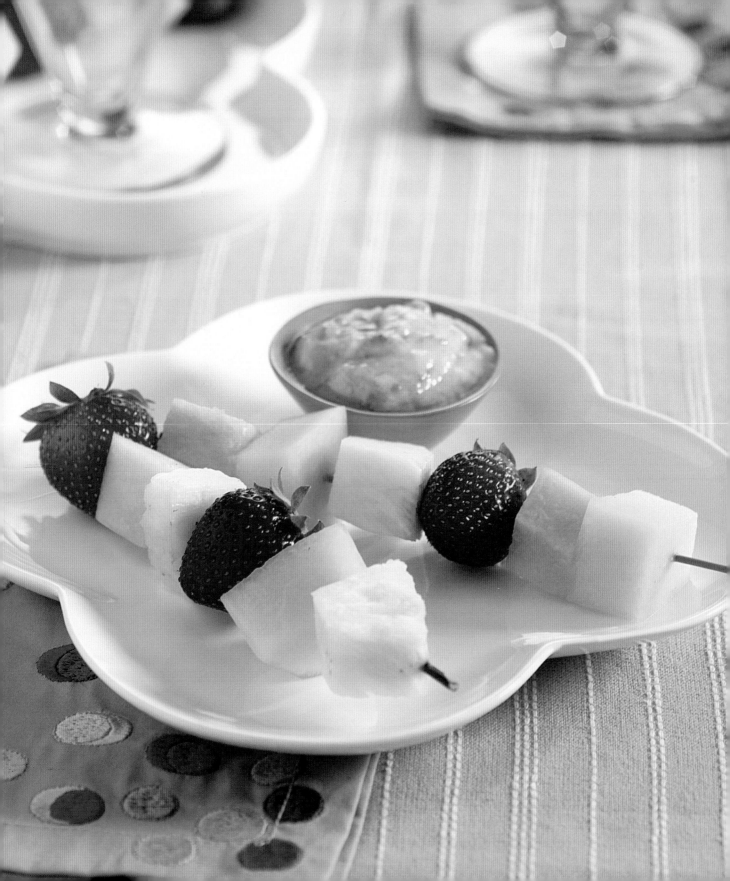

Chai Spiced Brown Rice & Chia Pudding

MAKES 4 TO 6 SERVINGS

- 4 **English breakfast tea bags**
- ½ **cup uncooked short grain brown rice, rinsed well**
- ¼ **cup chia seeds**
- ¼ **teaspoon ground cardamom**
- 1 **teaspoon ground cinnamon**
- ½ **teaspoon ground ginger**
- ¼ **teaspoon salt**
- 4 **cups almond milk**
- 2 **tablespoons maple syrup**
- ¼ **cup raisins**

1 Pour 1 cup boiling water into heat-safe mug. Add tea bags; steep 5 minutes; discard tea bags.

2 Combine tea, rice, chia seeds, cardamom, cinnamon, ginger, salt, milk and maple syrup in large saucepan over medium-high heat; bring to a boil. Reduce heat to low. Cook 1 hour 30 minutes, partially covered, until rice is tender and mixture is thick and creamy, stirring occasionally. Remove any film that appears on surface. Stir in raisins.

3 Serve warm or at room temperature.

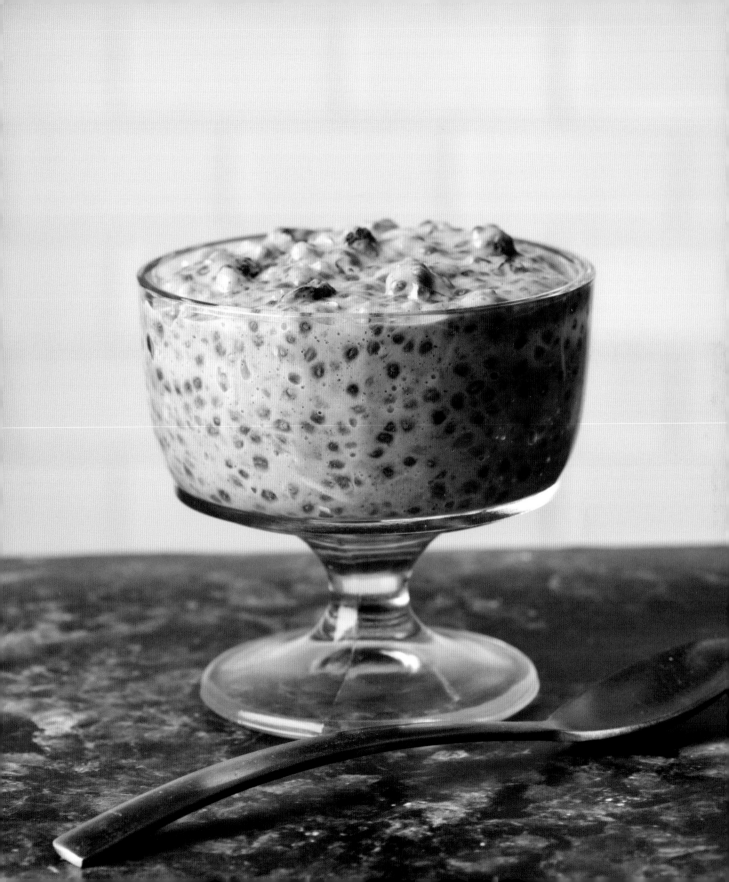

Chocolate Almond Truffles

MAKES 20 TRUFFLES (4 TRUFFLES PER SERVING)

½ **cup almond butter**

3 **tablespoons sugar substitute, such as stevia**

1 **cup crisp rice cereal**

3 **tablespoons unsweetened cocoa powder**

¼ **cup semisweet chocolate chips**

1 Place almond butter in small microwavable bowl. Microwave on HIGH 10 seconds. Stir in sugar substitute with wooden spoon until smooth. Stir in cereal; mix well.

2 Line large plate with waxed paper. Spray hands with nonstick cooking spray and shape mixture into 1-inch balls, pressing firmly. Place balls on prepared plate and freeze 15 minutes or up to 1 hour.

3 Spread cocoa on small plate. Roll each truffle in cocoa; return to large plate.

4 Place chocolate chips in small resealable food storage bag. Microwave on HIGH 10 seconds; knead bag. Repeat until chocolate is melted and smooth.

5 Press melted chocolate into one corner of bag; cut very small hole in corner. Drizzle chocolate over truffles. Let chocolate set before serving. Truffles can be refrigerated in airtight container up to 3 days.

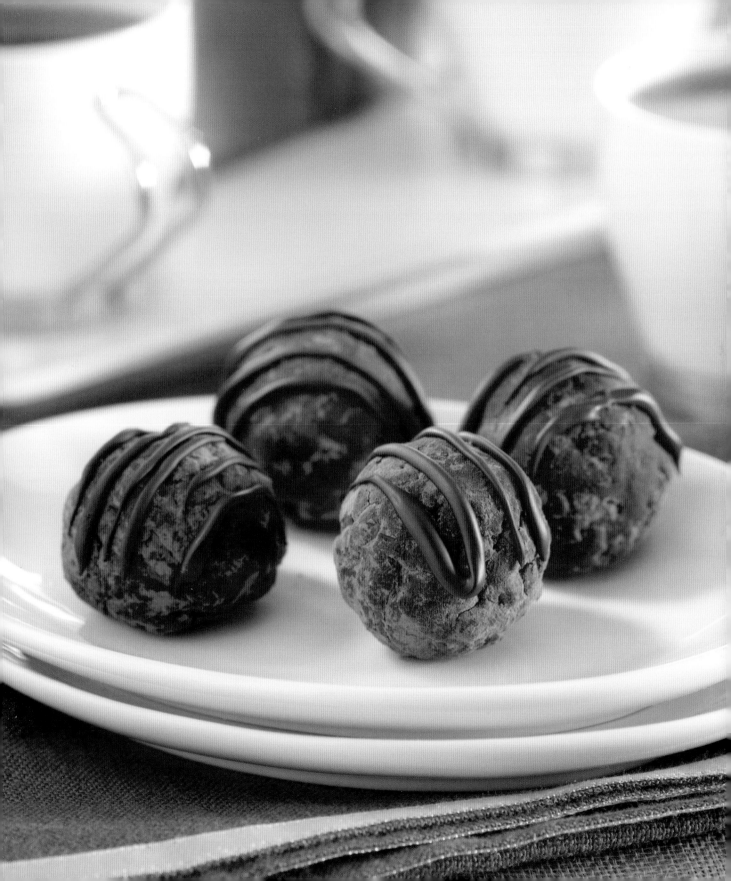

Banana & Chocolate Chip Pops

MAKES 4 SERVINGS

1 small ripe banana

1 container (6 ounces) plain nonfat Greek yogurt

⅛ teaspoon ground nutmeg

2 tablespoons semi-sweet chocolate chips

4 pop molds or paper cups and pop sticks

1 Slice banana; place in food processor. Add yogurt and nutmeg; process until smooth. Transfer to small bowl; stir in chips.

2 Spoon banana mixture into molds or cups. Set on level surface in freezer; freeze 2 hours or until firm. To unmold, briefly run warm water over molds until each pop loosens.

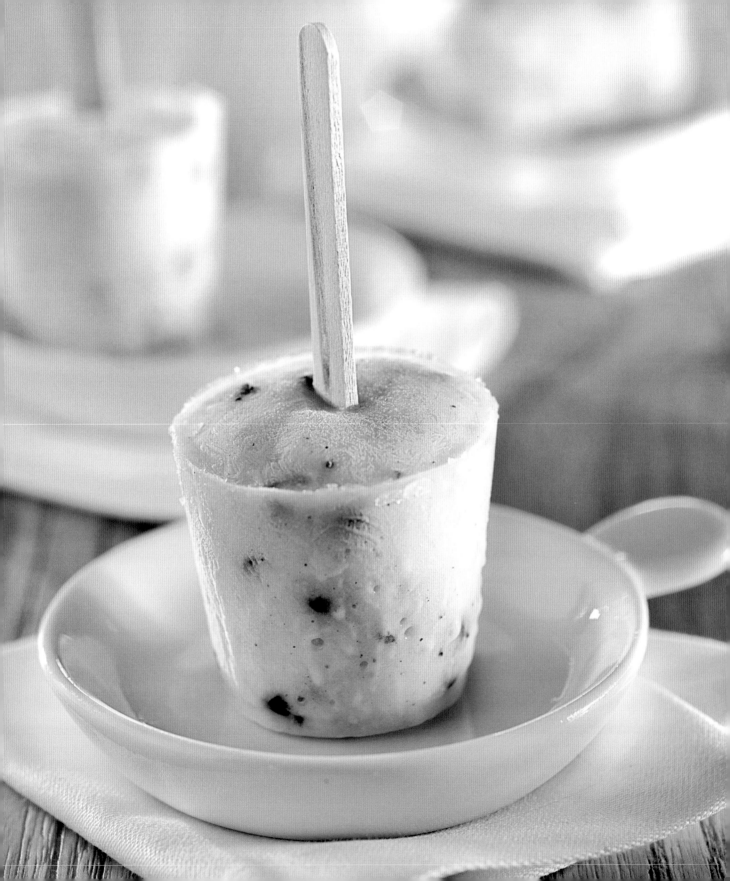

INDEX

INDEX

METRIC CONVERSION CHART

VOLUME MEASUREMENTS (dry)

1/8 teaspoon = 0.5 mL
1/4 teaspoon = 1 mL
1/2 teaspoon = 2 mL
3/4 teaspoon = 4 mL
1 teaspoon = 5 mL
1 tablespoon = 15 mL
2 tablespoons = 30 mL
1/4 cup = 60 mL
1/3 cup = 75 mL
1/2 cup = 125 mL
2/3 cup = 150 mL
3/4 cup = 175 mL
1 cup = 250 mL
2 cups = 1 pint = 500 mL
3 cups = 750 mL
4 cups = 1 quart = 1 L

VOLUME MEASUREMENTS (fluid)

1 fluid ounce (2 tablespoons) = 30 mL
4 fluid ounces (1/2 cup) = 125 mL
8 fluid ounces (1 cup) = 250 mL
12 fluid ounces (1 1/2 cups) = 375 mL
16 fluid ounces (2 cups) = 500 mL

WEIGHTS (mass)

1/2 ounce = 15 g
1 ounce = 30 g
3 ounces = 90 g
4 ounces = 120 g
8 ounces = 225 g
10 ounces = 285 g
12 ounces = 360 g
16 ounces = 1 pound = 450 g

DIMENSIONS

1/16 inch = 2 mm
1/8 inch = 3 mm
1/4 inch = 6 mm
1/2 inch = 1.5 cm
3/4 inch = 2 cm
1 inch = 2.5 cm

OVEN TEMPERATURES

250°F = 120°C
275°F = 140°C
300°F = 150°C
325°F = 160°C
350°F = 180°C
375°F = 190°C
400°F = 200°C
425°F = 220°C
450°F = 230°C

BAKING PAN SIZES

Utensil	Size in Inches/Quarts	Metric Volume	Size in Centimeters
Baking or Cake Pan (square or rectangular)	8×8×2	2 L	20×20×5
	9×9×2	2.5 L	23×23×5
	12×8×2	3 L	30×20×5
	13×9×2	3.5 L	33×23×5
Loaf Pan	8×4×3	1.5 L	20×10×7
	9×5×3	2 L	23×13×7
Round Layer Cake Pan	8×1½	1.2 L	20×4
	9×1½	1.5 L	23×4
Pie Plate	8×1¼	750 mL	20×3
	9×1¼	1 L	23×3
Baking Dish or Casserole	1 quart	1 L	—
	1½ quart	1.5 L	—
	2 quart	2 L	—